Embrace the journey
♡ Michelle

the YOU REVOLUTION®

the Journey of a Better Being

D1531330

MICHELLE ZELLNER

the YOU Revolution®: The Journey of a Better Being
Published by Pink Penny Publishing
Denver, CO

Copyright ©2019 Michelle Zellner. All rights reserved.

No part of this book may be reproduced in any form or by any mechanical means, including information storage and retrieval systems without permission in writing from the publisher/author, except by a reviewer who may quote passages in a review.

All images, logos, quotes, and trademarks included in this book are subject to use according to trademark and copyright laws of the United States of America.

ISBN: 978-0-578-47499-1
Health & Fitness / Healthy Living

Cover and Interior design by Victoria Wolf

QUANTITY PURCHASES: Schools, companies, professional groups, clubs, and other organizations may qualify for special terms when ordering quantities of this title. For information, email michelle@betterbeings.net.

The ideas contained in this book are based upon the experience and opinion of the author. Please consider your own needs and consult your trusted healthcare professional to help determine what choices are best for you.

All rights reserved by Michelle Zellner and Pink Penny Publishing
This book is printed in the United States of America.

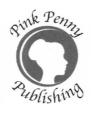

AUTHOR'S NOTE

Accounts of the events depicted in this book are factual.
The identities of some parties have been
changed to protect the guilty.

TABLE OF CONTENTS

PREFACE..7

INTRODUCTION......................................21
What Is Wellness?

CHAPTER ONE 29
Know Your Numbers

CHAPTER TWO 51
The Truth About Weight Loss

CHAPTER THREE 79
What Am I Supposed to Eat?

CHAPTER FOUR 103
Movement Is Medicine

CHAPTER FIVE 121
How's the Connection?

CHAPTER SIX.......................................149
Mind Matters—The Power of Thoughts

CHAPTER SEVEN....................................183
Balance Your Act

CHAPTER EIGHT....................................201
Are You Feeding Your Feelings?

CHAPTER NINE 219
Good Night Now!

CHAPTER TEN 237
Decades

REFERENCE SHEETS.................................245

PREFACE

ARE YOU READY TO MAKE your health a priority? Are you looking for ways to enhance your well-being? Have you recognized that something—maybe many things—have to change? If you answered yes to any or all of those questions, I invite you to be part of the YOU Revolution!

Before I tell you what the YOU Revolution is all about, let me tell you what it is NOT. It is not a diet. It is not a program. It is not a miracle, promising amazing things will happen overnight. It IS a journey of self-discovery, offering the chance to gain knowledge and develop strategies to make healthier choices in every aspect of your life. It is a starting point toward revolutionizing your well-being. This book is the product of the YOU Revolution 10-week class which I created and have been teaching since 2014, and it is also my story. Whatever topic I am teaching,

I like to approach it from a point of experience, and my personal journey has allowed me to share information that is relatable. If you have thought it, done it, or struggled with it, I have thought it, done it, or struggled with it—or I have worked with someone who has!

To help connect you to my message, and for topics discussed later in the book to make sense, I'd like to set you up with a little background information. My journey began in Winneconne, Wisconsin, population just under 2,000. My parents raised my sister and me to be independent, well-rounded kids, with certain expectations that were not negotiable. We were expected to work hard, focus on doing well in school, be kind, and love and respect each other. This was all done with sacrifice on their part and always with love, support, and encouragement. Still going strong, with fifty-two-plus years of marriage, my parents modeled the type of relationship everyone hopes for but few experience. To me, this was normal. I thought everyone had the same kind of parents I did, and I expected that someday I would enjoy a similar dynamic with a husband and family of my own.

At the age of seven, my friend's mom enrolled all of us (my sister, Nicolle; my friend Jesica her sister, Erin; and me) in a gymnastics class held at the University of Wisconsin–Oshkosh. This was about a thirty-minute drive from home, and each Tuesday and Thursday evening the four of us piled in the car, eager to go have fun. It was this exposure to gymnastics that set me up for many things that shaped my future self—some great, some not so great. Within one year I decided I wanted to be part of the "good group." That was a group of girls on the other side of the gym who were doing all kinds of amazing things that looked like a lot of fun. There were tryouts, and I made the cut. Jesica tells the story of how we all started out in gymnastics together, then she went away for the summer to visit her grandmother in Florida, and by the time she came back, I was doing tricks and flips. This was definitely the sport for me!

When I was in third grade, my parents took us on an incredible vacation to Hawaii. Now, by the age of eight, I was already a seasoned international traveler. My mother is from the Netherlands, so I had been to Europe a few times to visit my Oma and Opa. These visits were all prior to age five, and I have few, but vivid, memories. A small-town girl traveling to a foreign land was kind of a big deal, so it would seem like going to Hawaii, just another state, would not measure up. This trip, however, was life-changing for me. As we descended into the Honolulu airport, I felt like I was coming home. I can't explain it any other way than that. Being in the beautiful environment and feeling the aloha spirit all around felt normal and comfortable, like it was truly embedded in my soul. I knew from that point on that Hawaii would somehow be part of my life.

Recognizing common themes that run through one's life is an interesting discovery. They can go unnoticed for quite some time then, at a point of reflection, it all becomes very clear. One such theme in my life is feeling like I was never completely wanted and never quite belonged. Don't get me wrong; I was not an outcast or shunned, but just always on the fringe of the "cool club." Maybe the nugget was planted in my head because for a long time I did not really resemble any of my family members. A babysitter we had took that to a whole new level by telling me I was adopted. She actually told a story of how she saw my parents at an adoption agency in Chicago—according to her story that is how they met and why she is my babysitter. I had a recurring dream where my "mom" would show up at our front door holding a stack of packages in her arms.

She rang the doorbell because she needed help getting in. It was cold out and this person, "Mom," had on black leather gloves. I knew something wasn't right, because my mom would never wear those gloves. My sister was home in her room and heard me say something unusual so she called 911. I flew down our two flights of stairs and burst out the back door, running as fast and as far as I could. I saw police cars in the cornfield and they had my mom. This lady who showed up at the door was an imposter and wanted to take over our lives. Luckily, she did not know my sister was home and we were safe.

I recognized the correlation between this dream and being unsettled in my awake world, but I did not fully understand at the time how powerful my dreams were. The subconscious mind is always sending messages, and mine come through quite strongly while I am asleep. Throughout my life I have had warnings, answers, and ideas invade my peaceful nights. Eventually, I accepted this piece of me that I often found irritating, disturbing, and even sometimes scary. Tuning into my subconscious voice has become a rather significant factor in my journey, as embracing the messages in my dreams helped me push through some difficult times. Stay tuned for that story later in the book.

Getting back to the theme of "not belonging." Having a mom from a foreign country was odd in our little town. She would often speak Dutch in front of my friends, and it would really upset me. "Mom, we're in America—speak English!" I'd say. So she did, and she stopped speaking Dutch to me. This is definitely one of my regrets, as my entire family can speak and understand Dutch except for me. We lived out in the country, about five miles outside of Winneconne. It was an effort to go anywhere and for friends to visit, so it didn't happen often. In gymnastics, most of the girls on the team knew each other from schools in Oshkosh. At school, most of my friends became very close because of the bonds they forged on sports teams. When it came time for college, I spent my first two years at the University of Wisconsin-Oshkosh, and then completed my undergraduate education at the University of Hawaii-Manoa. I fulfilled my lifelong dream of living in Hawaii but again, this led to me not really belonging. I was a haole girl in a local world. Even though the essence of Hawaii lived in my soul, I was still a white girl from the mainland. Throughout my life, in my efforts to belong somewhere, I tried to belong everywhere. I wanted to be everyone's friend, no matter what clique they were part of. Sometimes it worked out well, sometimes not. In many cases I became a follower for no reason other than I wanted to be part of something. Perhaps you become good at what you are accustomed to, and this is how I developed an introverted nature. I don't know, but I do know that I've had to work very hard over the years to make sure I stay engaged with quality people and relationships. I've had to let go of ones that are not healthy or serve no real purpose so I can devote time and energy to the ones that really matter.

Once I arrived in Hawaii, where my physical being and my spirit could finally reside as one, I was ready to thrive. I had always loved travel and thought the hospitality industry was glamorous, so I entered the tourism management program. After one semester, I realized I hated it! Not really knowing what to do, I declared as a psychology major. I also thought I'd like to be a dietician, but biochemistry put a stop to that idea. My experience as a gymnast and my struggles with post-gym life often centered around an unhealthy relationship with food. I thought some nutrition classes might help me figure a few things out, so I loaded up on many of those as well. I went about getting my degree and rapidly realized I was going to have to do more, but again, I was not quite sure of the specifics. A year before I was due to graduate, I met David, who eventually became my fiancé. He was in the army stationed at Schofield Barracks and was the friend of my friend's husband. I was not ready to leave Hawaii after I graduated, as I had learned about the fantastic program for athletic training I knew this was right up my alley so I enrolled. Sadly, one semester after I started, they cut the program. Well, crap—now what? I decided going on for my master's degree was necessary, and sports psychology was the plan. I thought maybe I could utilize all my experience, skills, and knowledge to work with athletes with eating disorders. My two best friends from college, Kelly and Lisa, were both from Colorado. They convinced me that I must attend the University of Colorado Boulder, so I applied, was accepted, and was even granted a teaching assistant's position. This meant David and I would be enduring a long-distance relationship for at least one year until he could put in for a transfer, and, hopefully, get stationed at Fort Carson in Colorado Springs.

A few years before this, Kelly had landed back in Colorado and was scheduled to do her student teaching at a school just outside of Boulder. How perfect! I got to be roommates with one of my besties, and the little town of Gunbarrel was a great fit for us. As I settled into life as a graduate student, being in a committed long-distance relationship, I studied, worked, and worked out. That was basically my life. I found a great job working at the front desk of a health club in Gunbarrel, which was ideal. It offered me a free membership, access to everything the club had to offer, and plenty of time to study while I earned a bit of money. It was here that I was introduced to personal training. Keep in mind, this is 1996, before everyone and his cousin were personal trainers, before personal training was even a "thing." The trainer at the club—the only trainer at the club—was about to have a baby. She suggested I get certified and cover her clients while she was gone. I considered this a great opportunity and gave it a shot. Turned out, I loved it—and I was pretty good at it. It combined all of my passions: fitness, nutrition, and helping people. The money was not bad either. By the time she returned, I had a full slate of my own clients and knew this was the path I would take. We were independent contractors so I had to come up with a business name. What was my purpose—help people with their bodies, help people with their minds, help people become better human beings. Thus, my company Better Beings was born.

Just as I was hitting my stride professionally, I was wrapping up my education. David had been transferred, but rather than to Fort Carson, it was Fort Hood, Texas. I was not thrilled with the location, but we got engaged, and I left my thriving business to build a life with my future husband. Texas was hot. No, I mean HOT. The summer of 1998 was one of the hottest on record at the time, and the humidity! UGH! I had really embraced the dry climate of Colorado. OK, if I'm honest, it was all about the hair. My natural curls loved the dry climate. Oh, the things we do for love—like move to places nobody would generally volunteer to live. But here I was, in a new town, ready to get started. I did know one person—the friend whose husband is David's friend—they were also at Fort Hood. This was great—a friendly and familiar face was just what I needed. I ended up working at a gym she was working at and soon was building a client base. I also met Martha, a sassy lady a few years older than I was. She had a zing to her that I loved. It was a bit overbearing at times, but something about the way she carried herself and went about business really appealed to me. I knew I wanted to be her friend, and she embraced me immediately. After a brutally hot summer, working hard to set up a household, build a business, and plan a wedding, I got the first real shocking blow to my young heart. A girl from Hawaii called at two o'clock on a Friday afternoon asking for David. After a few questions I knew who she was—a fellow soldier from Schofield Barracks—and I asked her why she was calling. It went something like this:

Dana: Has David told you anything about me?

Me: Well, other than you know each other from base, no. Why? Is there something else I should know?

Dana: Well, we kind of messed around a while ago when

he was still here, and our son is turning one next month.
I just thought you should know that before
you married him.

Me: Come again?

OK . . . my reaction was a little different than that, but I'll let you fill in those details. Feeling very alone and shattered, my first phone call was to my bestie Kelly. I needed someone who knew me, knew David, and would offer nothing but comfort, and she did just that. David arrived home shortly after and our exchange is something I will never forget. The look of devastation on his face—at what he had done, how he had hurt me, how he had probably destroyed the best thing he ever had. It was quite sad on so many levels. "It" happened over Christmas break the previous year. He didn't want to spend the money to come home for Christmas so he stayed in Hawaii. That decision to not spend $800 on a plane ticket ended up costing him SO much more. We spent the next week going through every emotion you can imagine. In many ways it was the most incredible week we'd ever had together. I think sometimes that happens when you know your time is up. Making the phone call to my parents was one of the most difficult things I've ever done. Still to this day it ranks up there in the top three. I knew that once the call was made, and the story was told, there was no going back. I think I was most angry at David for the hurt this was going to cause my parents. I'm sure this is not what any parent wants for their child, especially one who sacrificed everything she had and did nothing to deserve it. The call was made. David and I spent a few days packing up, contemplating the future, and doing our best to be OK. Dad flew to Dallas, and I drove to pick him up. We then went on the twenty-hour drive back to Wisconsin, talking the whole way but saying nothing about the situation. When we rolled into the driveway of the house I grew up in—where I had not lived for many years—the flood gates opened. My mom was waiting in the driveway, and the tears poured down. I felt like a failure in so many ways. Here I was, twenty-six years old, thinking I had my future planned, and in an instant it all changed. The movie Sliding Doors is my all-time favorite. It is a movie of parallel lives. In one the girl just barely makes the train and in the parallel one she just misses it. We get to follow her life in each version all the way to the end. I spent many hours, days, years thinking about how different things would have been had he just bought the plane ticket. I came to the point where I knew what did happen most likely would have been the eventual outcome anyway, but it took me a long time to get there. Everything really does happen for a reason; often you just don't know what that reason is.

I am now in Wisconsin, heading into winter, having no clue what is next. The idea of people paying me to make them exercise is a bit of a foreign concept at this time in this place, but I found a club in Neenah—about a forty-minute drive— that was open to me hanging out my shingle. That's the good news. The bad news is my cut would be $14 an hour. In Colorado and Texas, I was charging $35–$45 a session, so this was tough to swallow. Still, it was the only option on the table. I did the best I could to plod along, put on a happy face, and try to be productive. By February of 1999, I knew Wisconsin was just not the place for me, and I was ready to move on. My parents were nothing but wonderful through all of this, but I was not born to live with Mom and Dad forever (although I'm pretty sure they would have loved it). Martha and I developed a tight friendship during our brief three months together, and she thought maybe Austin would be a good place for me. I loved that idea! It was a fun medium-size city and health oriented, and I knew I would do well as a personal trainer. Getting to live close to a great friend added to its appeal. I also had a lot of love and support from friends and former clients in Boulder, and I considered that as an option as well. I remember standing in the kitchen one evening telling my dad I had decided it was time to go, and I was thinking I'd head to either Austin or Boulder. The look of terror on his face when I said "Austin" was all I needed to make Boulder the final decision. You see, Austin is only forty-five minutes away from Fort Hood. During my time at home, David and I had been communicating via phone and email and were talking about trying to work things out. There was so much that was going to have to happen to make it work, but if he was willing to put in the effort, so was I. He was heading to do a stint in Bosnia, so it really didn't matter where I landed, but being that close to the scene of the crime probably wouldn't have been a great idea.

Upon my return to Boulder, I was greeted by the faces of many friends who offered love and support and a helping hand to reestablish myself. I was getting letters every day from David, but at the same time I was finding strength in being distanced. It was helpful to not be able to talk to him, and as my head cleared, so did the vision of what I wanted for my future. The bottom line is he lied to me, he cheated on me, and he has a child who isn't mine. This is too much when you haven't even really started your life together. It is not the standard my parents set for me, and it is not the standard I chose for myself. My sister and I took a three-week trip to Europe in May of that year, and this was the first time since leaving Texas that I had absolutely no contact with David. Three solid weeks to really think. I came home and sent him an email telling him there was no chance that it could work—it was over. I asked him to respect my decision and to not write me, call me, or email me—please do not ever contact me again. We both had a lot of healing to do and I felt it was best accomplished done separately. My request was honored, and after a time I once again found my place, hit my stride, and forged ahead.

My client load at the gym was growing and eventually Better Beings expanded to include in-home personal training. I marketed myself the old-fashioned way—hitting the pavement with my trifold flyers I made at home with Print Shop. Funny to think this is what marketing used to look like! I knew I was a fortunate one, earning a rather nice living doing something I absolutely loved. I met the most amazing people, many who are, to this day, still dear to my heart. They invited me into their homes, their lives, and their minds, and with many of them it became a reciprocal relationship. I had a new set of friends and surrogate families who were kind, generous, supportive, and helpful. Some gave valuable business advice, others provided encouragement, and all offered love. They were as much my cheerleaders as I was theirs. All the while, they were getting their butts whupped—because that is why they hired me! I knew I was helping to improve their lives, creating Better Beings. I was living my values and it felt amazing!

Throughout all of this, I was growing and transforming professionally. I got involved with corporate wellness providers, working at health fairs, and doing onsite biometric screenings. Several of my clients owned businesses and asked me to teach classes to their employees—something on nutrition, or lowering blood pressure, or how to fit exercise into their busy schedules. I discovered I really enjoyed creating the content and teaching it. I had a thirst for knowledge and became fascinated with how the human body functions and how the choices we make, or don't make, affect it. If I wondered about these things, I bet other people did too. My list of topics was growing, and I saw this as a new branch of opportunity for my business.

Over the next few years my business thrived, but personally I was becoming rather stagnant. I enjoyed the town of Gunbarrel, but it really is no place for a cool, single, thirty-something female. I was spending a lot of time driving to Denver to have fun and realized I needed a change of scenery—and fast! One weekend in the spring of 2003, I went to Denver with a few of my friends to enjoy a fabulous brunch at The Tattered Cover Café where a client of mine had just become the chef. My friend

Cindy and I loved looking at real estate, and as we passed a high-rise complex with the "MODEL OPEN" sign, we stopped in to check it out. After fiveminutes, I decided I was going to buy one. It was totally me and just where I needed to be. Cindy was a little freaked out at this decision and suggested I take some time to think about it. Not necessary—but I did need to figure out how I was going to pay for it! I owned the condo in Gunbarrel, as well as a rental property in Greeley, which left me with little money for the down payment. I didn't want to sell my place quite yet because I knew it would make a great rental, so my wonderful parents stepped in and provided a short-term loan. Here I went—off to live in the city! I have always been a city girl at heart, and this was the first time I finally got to live in one. I had a beautiful unit in a great complex with awesome amenities and no shortage of vibrant young people around me. This was going to be amazing! And it was, for a very long time.

Living downtown gave access to so many fun opportunities—concerts, baseball games, hockey games, incredible restaurants and nightclubs. I was single and having a blast. By this point, I didn't care if I stayed single the rest of my life. It wasn't my preference, but I'd rather be single forever than settle for less than what I wanted—what my parents had. Enter Travis. This guy changed my world in so many ways. It was ALL so totally unexpected, from start to finish. I won't get into the details (that's a whole other book), but the short version is we got married nine months after our first date. It was incredible and amazing, and then it wasn't. And then it REALLY wasn't. And then it still wasn't. My experience with David was nothing compared to what I went through with Travis. Everything about our time together served a purpose, and now, many years removed, the purpose is clear. Without Travis, I would not believe in the power of energy and sharing a connection on an energetic level with another human being. I have NO DOUBT that this is real. I would not be able to fully appreciate and empathize with someone who struggles with mental health issues. I would not be able to relate and provide guidance to individuals who have a loved one who struggles with mental health issues. I would not know what it really means to accept, forgive, and let go. I would not have grown to recognize the power of the subconscious that we tend to ignore. I would have had no need to build the compassion, strength, and character that are part of who I am today. Travis is why I am a Better Being. Do not misunderstand. He did not make me a Better Being. I had many difficult choices to make throughout our time together, and for many years after, we no longer had contact. I decided to make the healthy choices—the hard ones—and the amount of growth as a human being that came along with those hard choices resulted in a Better Being.

Having gone through this major shake-up of my life, I devoted all of my energy to work. I wanted to be busy so I had no time to think. This was a fantastic strategy, and business was exploding. In the spring of 2014, one of my professional contacts reached out to me about an idea she had for her clients. She was working with a group that had an employee wellness program and wanted to offer something to help people improve their lifestyle habits. She asked if I was interested, and oh, by the way, they want to start in three weeks. Yes, yes, a thousand times, yes! I loved a challenge, especially now. I considered all the things that are required to make a healthy human being. I reflected on the things I have learned along the way, from the textbook information during my education to my own challenges and how I worked through them. I developed the ten-week class known as the YOU Revolution.

Having taught the class for many years, and witnessing how it has positively impacted the lives of hundreds of people, I decided it was time to write the book. I have stories to share, many you may recognize as your own. They are not always easy stories to tell, to open up and expose some of the yucky realities of life, but I know many people have found themselves in similar situations and have similar challenges. My hope in writing this book is to offer insight, ideas, guidance, and solutions to make your journey a little easier, and at the very least to let you know you are not alone.

We are all human beings . . . let's all be Better Beings.

Introduction

WHAT IS WELLNESS?

FOR MUCH OF MY LIFE, wellness centered around diet, exercise, and my weight. If I fit into my jeans, I was WELL! As I navigated through life, enduring some rather difficult experiences, I realized that wellness embodies so much more than that. I began to seriously contemplate what "wellness" meant to me when I was approached about creating the lifestyle change class that ultimately became *the You Revolution*. I had already gone through a bit of a metamorphosis of my lifestyle, becoming more engaged in habits that allowed me to lose weight (and finally keep it off), have more energy, and get better sleep. Central to all of this was my mindset of truly embracing the notion that what happens in our minds dictates what comes next—from a thought to a feeling to an energy and finally to an action.

The concept of wellness looks different depending on who you ask. For one person it may mean the absence of disease, and another may define wellness as having the strength and energy to keep up with the grandkids. What is your vision of wellness? Once you have defined it, you can then determine how close you are to living well. When I think about what wellness really looks like to me, it is the sum of a whole bunch of parts—my health status, what I put in my body, how much I move my body, how I manage my stress, how much sleep I am getting, the strength and value of relationships I have, and what my internal dialogue sounds like. If I am making healthy choices in all of those areas more often than not, I am well.

What is your definition of wellness? Create your vision of that definition, assess how close you are to it, and what you need to do to get closer. This is the beginning of *the You Revolution*—your journey to becoming a Better Being. I am a big believer in the value of getting thoughts out of our heads and into the real world, and I encourage you to make a vision board that depicts exactly what life will look like when you are well. Grab a piece of poster board, some magazines, and scissors, then glue and assemble pictures, words, and phrases that embody your idea of your healthy self living the life you desire. Use this as your guide, your inspiration, and your motivation for making those hard choices that will allow you to achieve the outcome you say you want. Decide today to no longer be a bystander but an active participant in your own life. It is going to be hard. That's right—healthy choices are hard! The world we live in does not make it easy because the unhealthy choices are almost always more convenient, more fun, more entertaining, and sometimes less expensive. That's why we often keep making the unhealthy choice. If the healthy choice was always the easy choice, there would be no book to write. I say, pick your hard. Eating healthy is hard—diabetes is harder. Exercising is hard—missing out on life because you don't have the stamina to live it is harder. Losing weight is hard—being fat is harder. Letting go is hard—going through life angry and bitter is harder. Pick your hard.

There are multiple dimensions of wellness, and the journey of a Better Being requires growth and change in all of them. *the You Revolution* is structured to allow you to identify what dimensions you need to address, including various aspects of physical, mental, and emotional health. Each of the following chapters is designed to offer insight, understanding, and practical tools to apply in your life. Start at the beginning or jump into a section that speaks to you. It is YOUR journey and you are in charge of the route you take.

THE INSIDE STORY

Do you know your numbers? When was the last time you had a full checkup with complete lab work? How do you feel? The body tries to tell us a lot, but we tend to ignore it or are so consumed with other things, we don't even hear it! The "Know Your Numbers" chapter is devoted to taking a deep dive into the numbers you should know, what they actually mean, and what lifestyle habits you may be engaging in that could be putting you at risk for suboptimal functioning and chronic disease.

IT'S A HEAVY ISSUE

Have you achieved and been able to maintain a healthy weight? Do you even know what a "healthy" weight is? "The Truth About Weight Loss" is a well-rounded investigation into what it takes to lose weight, and more important, keep it off! I pull no punches and keep it real. You may not like what I have to say, but I promise once you have the tools for success, your own revolution will be under way.

NUTRITION IN A NUTSHELL

Ask ten people what it means to "eat healthy," and you'll get ten different answers. Nutrition is a personal choice, but there are some basic tenets that apply to almost everyone. When you finish the chapter "What Am I Supposed to Eat?," you will have the guidelines necessary for you to determine what a "healthy diet" looks like for you. Do not gloss over this chapter, as I will reveal life-changing information. It is a discovery I made that has truly allowed me to be a Better Being, and I can't wait for you to join the party.

ARE YOU REALLY EXERCISING?

I have always believed exercise is the magic pill for everything—you just have to do it, almost every day, and for your whole life. "Movement Is Medicine," and this chapter will be your guide to embracing it as a necessary fact of life. I know, I know—you don't like to exercise, you don't have time, it's too hot, you're too tired. I have just the prescription for you, and if you swallow it, you will enjoy the amazing benefits exercise has to offer.

CAN YOU HEAR ME NOW?

We know that positive social connections and healthy relationships are necessary to thrive. The "How's the Connection?" chapter is intended to remind you of this. Because of the dominant role technology plays, I touch on the implications of overuse and how this can significantly impact physical, mental, and emotional well-being as well as interpersonal relationships. You also will be introduced to many of the personal relationships I've had throughout my life and the valuable lessons learned that spurred major growth in my own journey.

BUCKLE UP—THIS ONE'S BUMPY

Do you believe in the power of thoughts? When someone would tell me to change my attitude, my usual reaction was an eye roll. The "Mind Matters" chapter brings you into parts of my life that were a bit complicated. I will share experiences—some from this world and even some from another—that played key roles in shaping my future. This transformation occurred late in my journey and was by far the most difficult task, but harnessing thoughts and choosing what to do with them is absolutely the nucleus of being a Better Being.

STRESSED?

Anyone? No, seriously, are you? Of course you are. We all have stress, and the problem is, it's killing us. We all are exposed to potential stressors on a daily basis, and although it is unrealistic to think you can eliminate stress from your life, knowing how to manage it can make the difference between mental and physical productivity and detrimental health consequences. "Balance Your Act" is an interactive chapter with worksheets and assessments to help highlight why you are out of balance and demonstrate how to live in alignment with your goals, values, and priorities.

FOOD FOR THOUGHTS

What is your relationship with food? For many, it's a love/ hate relationship . . . a best friend and the worst enemy. "Are You Feeding Your Feelings?" explores all the reasons we eat, why we choose certain foods at certain times, and how this can lead to a life of struggle with health, weight, and self-esteem. You may even discover that although you think you are making a healthy choice, you might actually be setting yourself up for "caving in" to the forbidden food. Great news—I am an expert at food for therapy and am here to share the secrets to success for overcoming emotional eating.

SLEEP—IT DOES A BODY GOOD

According to the National Sleep Foundation, nearly 75 percent of all adults have trouble sleeping on more than two nights per week. We are a chronically sleep-deprived nation, and it's not working out well! As someone who has often found quality sleep difficult to come by, I know the impact our daily habits have on our ability to rest. In "Good Night Now!" I share the discoveries

I have made along my journey and will convince you that sleep is NOT a luxury but a necessity if you really want to be a Better Being.

TIME IS FLYING

"Decades" is the final chapter of the book, but it is nowhere near the end of your journey, for in life, there are no breaks. We all know time flies and this chapter will outline things you should be aware of from your thirties to sixties. It is an overview, revisiting previous themes, providing reminders of important concepts, and possibly challenging you to new levels. It is never too late (or early) to make changes in your habits and reap the benefits. Get started now so you have the rest of your life to enjoy them!

So once again I ask, "What is wellness?" Has your idea changed since the start of this introduction? I have taught hundreds of wellness classes to thousands of people, heads nodding in agreement with my words and stories, only to have people walk out the door and do nothing about it. *the You Revolution* is different. At the end of each chapter I will give you things to consider. In my onsite classes these are affectionately called homework. They are simply concepts outlined in each chapter, that, when applied in your daily life, will move you toward a Better Being. Your first tasks are, should you choose to embark on the revolution:

1. Create your personal wellness definition. If you have a family, come up with a family mission statement.

2. Identify any areas where you know change is necessary to achieve an outcome you are striving for.

3. Create a vision board that embodies your vision of wellness.

FINAL THOUGHTS

I just gave you a whole bunch of things to think about, and you may be feeling overwhelmed. Analysis paralysis will lock you down right where you are, so don't worry about where to start—just pick a chapter and start! Get out of all-or-nothing thinking. Pick one thing and be patient with the process. This is a journey. Change does not happen overnight and does not happen because you hoped it would. It is hard, uncomfortable, and sometimes messy. The instant result with no effort is NOT REALITY. Embrace the process and go forth with an open mind, kind heart, and the reminder of WHY you are doing it. After all, that's what a Better Being does.

Chapter One

KNOW YOUR NUMBERS

YOUR INSIDE NUMBERS TELL A story, and although no single number tells you much of anything, looking at all of them together, and how they are playing with each other, can tell you a lot. I was introduced to biometric screenings back in 1997 well before onsite wellness was a thing. I worked at a health club, both as a personal trainer, and at the front desk, while putting myself through graduate school. One of our members was talking about a health fair at his company and suggested I be part of the team who conducted the screenings. I honestly hadn't the slightest clue as to what he was talking about, but he gave me the contact information of the person in charge and off I went. Onsite wellness screenings soon became a solid source of income, and I became well versed in all aspects of the process, including blood pressure, cholesterol profile, glucose tests, BMI, and waist circumference. I often was the "health coach," designated to interpret results with the client and offer suggestions on how to improve their numbers. I became fascinated with thoroughly understanding what all these numbers mean, why they are important, and most important, how the choices we make regularly impact them. I wanted to know more—not simply that the choices have an impact, but how and why they have an impact. It drove me to educate myself further so I could explain, on a level everyone could understand, how the human body responds to things we do—or do not do—on a regular basis.

In the early 2000s, onsite wellness was taking off, with more and more companies providing these screenings for employees. I had the opportunity to visit the same companies and see the same people as in previous years. Over time, I saw many people change the direction of their health by changing their habits. I have witnessed people get off blood pressure medication, reverse the course of their diabetes, and shed the weight that was preventing them from living a fulfilling life. It is so empowering to know that you are in control of your health! I am going to coach you in the next few pages to help you understand the numbers, understand what you may be doing that is putting your numbers into an unhealthy range, and give you ideas on how to go about modifying behaviors for a happy inside story.

Ultimately, these numbers aid in assessing your level of disease risk, which basically comes down to hormonal balance and the health of your heart and arteries. The numbers I encourage you to know will provide the outline and help determine in what direction your health is headed.

HORMONES RULE

Hormones literally rule your world. I will be talking about hormones a lot throughout the book, so I want to briefly lay a foundation. When you hear the word "hormones," what comes to mind? Puberty . . . menopause . . . 'roid rage? If this describes your reaction, I want you to erase those thoughts and start over. There is so much more to hormones than just estrogen and testosterone. The body functions utilizing a complex system of these chemicals, which are basically messengers that tell every system what to do. Humans have fifty different types of hormones, many produced by the endocrine system. Some are very specific to the mechanisms they are in charge of, and others have their fingers in everything. One of the keys to optimal physical and mental well-being is hormonal balance.

I cannot possibly cover every duty of every hormone (nor do I profess to know every duty of every hormone), but I am going to highlight a few of the VIPs.

Insulin

You may think of diabetes when you hear the word "insulin." True, it is a key player in that disease, but insulin is just one of the blood sugar-regulating hormones. It is produced by the pancreas and released into the bloodstream when glucose is detected. Its job is to get glucose, the form of sugar used by the body, out of the bloodstream and into the cells. Once the cells have fuel, they can proceed to carry out their specific duties. Where we get into trouble is if we over-fuel, don't use our fuel, or don't fuel ourselves in the proper way. Achieving and maintaining steady blood sugar is another key to optimal physical and mental well-being. It is easy to get off track, but I will share all the secrets to keeping it steady!

Leptin and Ghrelin

I love these critters! So many things in my life made sense once I learned about leptin and ghrelin—the hunger hormones. Leptin is produced in fat cells and released to signal satiety. Ghrelin is the growler, produced in the lining of the stomach to signal you need to eat. Understanding these two hormones, specifically, what causes them to get out of balance, changed my life. I can't wait to share this information with you! There is no practical lab test to identify levels of leptin and ghrelin, but with the information in this book you will have a good idea if yours may be out of balance.

Cortisol

You might recognize cortisol as the "stress" hormone, gaining lots of attention in recent years. I like to think of cortisol as our survival hormone, because without it we would not be here today. You are going to get to know cortisol quite well as you read each chapter, because it is the boss! It dictates the roles of certain functions and of other hormones. You can test cortisol levels in a variety of ways. The saliva or urine tests are the most reliable. Kits can be ordered online or through your doctor.

TSH

Thyroid-stimulating hormone is probably one of the least understood hormones. I have become fascinated with learning more about thyroid functioning and the various thyroid hormones, because these messengers are in direct control of nearly everything—heart rate, blood pressure, body temperature, and metabolism, just to name a few. I will cover TSH in the "Balance Your Act" chapter, but this is such a complicated system that I encourage you to read *Stop the Thyroid Madness*, by Janie A. Bowthorpe, M.Ed. This book has led me to a much greater understanding of the challenges with diagnosing an underperforming thyroid system, which could possibly be the key to unlocking the mysteries surrounding your health issues. I think we should all have FULL thyroid panel testing, but unfortunately your regular doctor is probably not well versed in this area and you will receive either insufficient testing, inadequate interpretation, or improper diagnoses. Please arm yourself with as much knowledge as possible before approaching your doctor with the suggestion to have your thyroid tested, then be your own advocate. You may be dismissed, ignored, belittled, misguided, angered, and frustrated. Remember, you are the customer and the doctor works for you! If the doctor says you are just fine and you don't need those tests, I encourage you to push back and demand them. Bring a copy of the book with the pertinent information highlighted and invite your doctor to read it so you can navigate these waters together. If there is an unwillingness to address your concerns, a new doctor might be the best medicine. It may be a long, difficult process to find the right one who will treat you properly, but it will be worth it. Your physical, mental, and emotional health—your life—could depend on it!

Testosterone, Estrogen, Progesterone

These are not male hormones and female hormones; they are human hormones! We all have them and we all need them—ideally at optimal and balanced levels. The roles of these sex hormones are vast, and as the production of them declines with age, many aspects of physical and mental well-being also decline. As is the case with many medical discoveries, the results of one research study can lead us in a horribly wrong direction. Such was the fate of estrogen and hormone replacement therapy. We have now been taught to fear these hormones, assigning blame to them for everything from heart disease to cancer. The reality is that our sex hormones protect us. They keep us young and vibrant and free of disease. I highly recommend you read the book *How to Achieve Healthy Aging*, by Dr. Neal Rouzier. He makes it easy to understand exactly why we need each of these hormones, and why we should not fear them. He outlines how and WHY we were so misguided in our attitude and beliefs about the roles estrogen, testosterone, and progesterone play in men and women. There is also great information about DHEA and melatonin, two other key players in many body functions. I am convinced that when you understand how the body works, you too will be a believer in the value of properly balanced, optimal hormone levels. Getting these levels tested could provide the answers to many of the frustrations you may be struggling with surrounding your health. As with the case of thyroid functioning, your primary doctor may not be on board with testing or have adequate knowledge of how and why to properly treat. Again, I say arm yourself with knowledge, prepare for the fight, and be your own advocate.

Now that I have told you a few things your doctor may not be able to help you with, here are the things he or she probably hounds you about. And, yes, it is also important information you should have.

BLOOD PRESSURE—KEEP IT LOW

Maintaining healthy blood pressure is one of the best things you can do to enhance your quality of life and reduce your risk for all diseases. Your arteries are the transportation system delivering oxygen and nutrition to all organs and muscles. Hypertension, or chronic high blood pressure, causes damage to the arteries and over time can have a significant effect on your body's ability to function optimally. Understanding the risks associated with hypertension and how to prevent it will enable you to make lifestyle improvements. If left unchecked, serious consequences may lie ahead.

Hypertension

Blood pressure is the amount of force on your artery walls during the contraction and resting phases of your heartbeat. High blood pressure, or hypertension, indicates higher than normal pressure on the artery walls. The force of blood being pumped, amount of blood going through the arteries, and size and flexibility of your arteries all play a role in blood pressure.

Sometimes referred to as the silent killer, hypertension has no symptoms or warning signs. It is estimated that one-third of those with hypertension do not even know! Ideal blood pressure is 120/80 or less. Although there are several categories of hypertension, anything higher than 120/80—or either number being out of range—puts you in a risk category. Those with blood pressure of 140/90 or greater are at significantly increased risk for heart disease, stroke, and memory loss.

Because you don't feel hypertension, it can be easily ignored. The only way to know is by having your blood pressure checked regularly. Blood pressure can fluctuate throughout the day, so it is a good idea to check it at various times and following different types of situations. This will help you identify if lifestyle changes are necessary.

The Numbers

SYSTOLIC
(120) | TOP NUMBER
Force during heart contraction
Higher degrees of variation is acceptable

DIASTOLIC
(80) | BOTTOM NUMBER
Force during relaxation phase
Should be more constant

PULSE PRESSURE
Difference between systolic and diastolic
Ideally no more than 40
>40 may indicate blocked or rigid arteries

LEFT VS. RIGHT
Have both checked!
Despite health professionals routinely saying it doesn't matter, how do you know if you never check! The reading on both sides should be similar, but a dramatic difference may indicate blocked or rigid arteries.

Some ups and downs are normal. We get a spike of adrenaline and a release of cortisol first thing in the morning, which increases our blood pressure and helps get us moving. For most people, blood pressure is highest at work and should dip while at home. Obviously, this depends on your stressors and how you handle them! In addition, exercise, caffeine, and medication (both prescription and over-the-counter [OTC]) can cause a spike in blood pressure. When you know your blood pressure and how it responds in these situations, you can take steps to minimize your risk of an event.

Age, race, and gender are things we can't change, but these factors have an effect on our risk. As we get older, body parts naturally wear out. How well you take care of yourself will largely determine how much damage occurs over time. African-American, Hispanic, and Native American populations all have a greater risk of hypertension; Caucasian and Asian populations have lower risk. Men are at double the risk of women, but after menopause the risk to women and men is nearly equal. The hormone estrogen plays a role in blood pressure regulation, which accounts for this factor. Although there is a genetic component to everything, just because there is family history of hypertension doesn't necessarily mean it is genetic. You have to look at the choices being made. If you are doing all the right things and still have high blood pressure, that IS genetic. Quite often, however, hypertension is due to unhealthy lifestyle choices.

Poor Stress Management

Stress is part of life, and although we can take steps to minimize it, managing it in a healthy way is important! In addition to increasing blood pressure itself, chronic stress can lead to behaviors that increase blood pressure. People often turn to unhealthy foods and alcohol to cope with stress while not taking time to do things that lower blood pressure naturally, like exercise, meditation, and getting adequate sleep.

Weight

The more you are carrying around, the harder your heart has to work. It is also possible that the extra weight is due to an unhealthy diet and not enough exercise—two additional factors that can affect your blood pressure.

Unhealthy Diet

Too much processed food and not enough real food can put you at risk for high blood pressure. The body was made to function on certain combinations of nutrients that are best found in real food. In particular, the minerals potassium, magnesium, calcium, and sodium work with each other to keep blood pressure regulated. The typical American diet is too high in sodium and deficient in potassium, magnesium, and calcium. Eating a wide variety of fruits, vegetables, nuts, whole grains, low-fat dairy, and lean protein will most likely provide your body with the necessary resources. And, if you are eating real food more often, you are probably minimizing the packaged, processed, and restaurant foods that are loaded with sodium. Aim to keep sodium under 2,400 mg/day (<1,500 if you have high blood pressure).

No amount of alcohol is good for people with high blood pressure. Three or more drinks causes a temporary spike, and chronic indulging can damage arteries and have lasting effects. In addition, alcohol can interfere with and decrease the effectiveness of blood pressure medications.

Consuming sugary foods or white refined carbohydrates can impact your blood pressure. Sugar in the blood triggers your pancreas to release insulin. This is normal and necessary, but when insulin is released, the blood reabsorbs sodium. If you are eating too much sugar, this can lead to too much sodium in the bloodstream. An excessive proportion of sodium to other minerals (potassium, magnesium, calcium) triggers an increase in blood pressure.

Fiber slows the rate at which sugar processes in the blood-stream. Aim for 14 g per 100 lb. of your body weight. A wide variety of fruits, vegetables, whole grains, and beans will ensure adequate fiber intake.

Caffeine triggers a release of cortisol, which, in turn, elevates heart rate and blood pressure. Other stimulants, including nicotine, taurine, and guarana extract, act in the same fashion. Some medications and OTC drugs also have stimulating effects.

BLOOD SUGAR—KEEP IT STEADY!

From the time you get up to the time you go to bed, steady blood sugar is critical for a healthy, successful day. It is key for maintaining your energy level, curbing cravings, keeping metabolism boosted, and improving focus and mental clarity. Spikes and crashes in blood sugar wreak havoc on hormonal balance, which is why steady blood sugar also plays a major role in achieving a healthy weight and in preventing disease!

To truly appreciate how blood sugar affects all of your body's systems, let's look at exactly how it works. Hormones regulate every process in our bodies, and glucagon and insulin are the two hormones that regulate our blood sugar levels. When we eat food, it gets broken down into glucose—the form of sugar the body uses. With glucose in the blood, a message is sent to the pancreas to release insulin. Insulin is responsible for getting glucose out of the blood and into the cells for your body to use. What doesn't get used gets sent to the liver for storage and gets metabolized into triglycerides to be stored in the body's fat cells. When blood sugar levels get low, glucagon sends a message to the liver to release stored glucose into the bloodstream.

We are very much in control of our blood sugar levels. What we eat, how much we move, the stress management tools we employ, and how much sleep we get all have an impact on our blood sugar regulation.

Diet

The first point to remember is that there is no ONE food that is bad for you and no food that has magic powers. We have to look at the whole picture when making food choices, including how it will affect blood sugar. Because refined carbohydrates and sugary foods leave very little for your body to break down, they cause an immediate spike in blood sugar, which is followed by the crash. Limit these foods and incorporate foods higher in protein, fiber, and fat. In fact, every time you eat a snack or a meal, you should have a combination of protein, fat, and fiber (a form of carbohydrate). A 40-30-30 percentage ratio of carbohydrates to protein to fat has been shown to be the ideal ratio for keeping blood sugar steady. That can be a lot of tedious math, so keep it simple by identifying a high-fiber carbohydrate, lean protein, and healthy source of fat each time you eat.

The Glycemic Index ranks foods from 1–100, measuring how quickly a food enters and exits the bloodstream. A food with a 100 spikes blood sugar; a food with a 1 has almost no effect on blood sugar. Keep in mind, just because one food has a lower number than another food doesn't mean it is better for you. Fat is something that slows down the absorption of sugar. A piece of chocolate cake could have a lower GI than a banana—but is cake better for you than a banana? IF ONLY!!

Exercise

The body's primary source of fuel is glucose. When we don't use it regularly, over time it stays elevated in the bloodstream. Moving your body every day will enable you to maintain insulin sensitivity—meaning your cells are responsive to insulin's instruction to open up and accept the fuel. When you lose this sensitivity, diabetes is the result.

By now most of us have heard about the importance of getting in 10,000 steps a day. There really is no magic to this number—that is just how much we are supposed to be moving because we are human. If you have a sedentary job, your first priority is to "get human." Dedicated exercise is also necessary to help manage blood sugar. Exercising at 65–85 percent of your Maximum Heart Rate utilizes blood sugar, blood fats, then stored fat. Ideally, we are exercising every day, but most important is to focus on doing as much as you can, as hard as you can, as often as you can.

Stress

A necessary reaction of the stress response, aka fight or flight, is to provide the body with extra available fuel to respond to a perceived threat. In the acute phase, this is critical to survival. In addition to extra blood sugar, we have extra fatty acids and higher levels of insulin, adrenaline, and cortisol. If stress is not managed properly, the acute turns chronic, leaving hormones out of balance and blood sugar chronically elevated.

Exercise is one of the healthiest stress management tools as it reverses many of the negative effects of chronic stress. Healthy nutrition is also critical as it can prevent further spikes in blood sugar and promote a steady release of glucose, insulin, and glucagon. Other tools that reestablish the mind-body connection, such as yoga, meditation, visualization, and deep breathing, are also healthy coping strategies. They lower cortisol levels and can reduce blood pressure by up to 10 points.

Sleep

Regulated by the hormones, glucagon and insulin, blood sugar levels rise and fall during waking and sleeping hours. Levels elevate in the evening and peak 3–4 hours after you fall asleep. If you are not getting deep, restful sleep or going through enough sleep cycles, these hormones, as well as many others, get thrown out of balance. Ghrelin is a hormone that signals your brain that you are hungry. Sleep deprivation leads to higher levels of ghrelin as well as depressed levels of leptin, the one that signals you are satiated. Less than adequate sleep also keeps blood sugar elevated, putting you right into the sugar cycle. A dedicated choice of protein and fat in the morning can help break this cycle and get your system back on track for hormonal balance.

CHOLESTEROL—KEEP IT CLEAN!

There seems to be a lot of confusion surrounding the topic of cholesterol. What do all the numbers mean? Does having high cholesterol really increase the risk for heart disease? Where does cholesterol come from and how much control do you have over your levels? Research is never ending, but we do have answers to these questions, and many more. The role cholesterol plays in our health—both positive and negative—is complex. The good news is the solutions to achieving healthy cholesterol levels and decreasing your risk for disease are fairly simple!

Cholesterol is a wax-like, fatty substance that is involved in many important functions in the body. Not only is it the structural component of cells, but it also is required for proper brain functioning. We need cholesterol to convert vitamin D into a form the body can use, produce hormones, and form bile, which is needed for digestion.

Generally, the liver produces all the cholesterol an individual needs—about 1,000mg per day. If you have "high" cholesterol, either your liver is overproducing it or it is a function of lifestyle choices. Eating too many of the wrong foods or not enough of the right foods and not being physically active are just a few of the ways daily habits influence cholesterol levels.

Knowing your numbers is an important first step toward reducing your risk for heart disease. The Lipid Profile test is a basic blood panel that will tell you Total Cholesterol, HDL, LDL, and Triglycerides; these are the levels to aim for:

Total Cholesterol <200
HDL >60
LDL <100
VLDL <30
TRG <150

The Lipid Profile is a good start and can indicate red flags, but at some point you may want to consider a more comprehensive Vertical Auto Profile (VAP) test. It turns out that size really does matter, and the VAP test breaks down the various sizes and densities of the cholesterol molecules. This information is particularly helpful if you have out-of-healthy-range levels or have family history of heart disease or diabetes.

HDL—The Good Stuff!

High-Density Lipoprotein molecules are the smallest cholesterol molecules, but they are very hard workers! They act as trash collectors in the bloodstream by grabbing on to LDL and transporting it to the liver for elimination. This helps keep arteries clear for maximum blood flow. HDL2, the larger type of HDL (vs. HDL3) is actually the one doing all the hard work. Research is showing that HDL3 offers no protection from heart disease. This is one example of how knowing more than just your total HDL level could be valuable information.

LDL—Lousy for Life!

Made up mostly of cholesterol with a little bit of protein and triglycerides, Low-Density Lipoprotein molecules are thought to be the ones that really increase the risk for heart disease. There are several subclasses of LDL, and levels of these all play a role in how great the risk may be.

A—larger, less dense, easy to remove
A/B—light and dense combo
*B—small and dense
*four times greater risk of developing heart disease

VLDL—Very Low-Density Lipoprotein

Mostly triglycerides with minimal protein, elevated levels of VLDL correspond to an increased risk of developing heart disease and diabetes.

Intermediate-Density Lipoprotein (IDL)
Formed from the degradation of VLDL
Contributes to atheroma
(an abnormal fatty deposit in an artery)
Family history of diabetes correlates to higher IDL

Lp(a)
Molecularly similar to LDL
Strong genetic factor
Most significant indicator of risk for heart attack

VLDL3
Smallest, most dense type of LDL
Difficult for HDL to bind and remove
Easiest to collect in artery walls
Increased risk for heart disease and diabetes

Triglycerides—Free-Floating Fat

Unlike HDL and LDL, these molecules have no protein component. Triglycerides are a source of fuel, but too much hanging out in the bloodstream can narrow the artery passage and cause a blockage. This leads to an increased risk for heart attack or stroke.

There are other subclasses of cholesterol that may prove to be critical in determining risk for disease.

Family history of heart disease or diabetes does put you in a risk category, but knowing the lifestyle habits of those family members is also important information. If it is a truly genetic condition, medication (in addition to healthy choices!) may be necessary to get your cholesterol to a healthy level. For most people, the habits we engage in over the course of time are the most profound factors either increasing or decreasing our risk for heart disease.

Nutrition

Unhealthy food—too much, too often, or for too long—can contribute to unhealthy cholesterol levels. Minimize low-quality fat, refined sugars, and alcohol, and eliminate trans fats altogether! Increase your fiber intake to help flush LDL and incorporate healthy fats to preserve HDL levels.

Exercise

Cardio exercise stimulates the liver to produce more HDL. In addition, it increases the size and density of HDL. Intensity, duration, and consistency are all necessary to achieve the desired effect. Remember the prescription:

DO AS MUCH AS YOU CAN, AS HARD AS YOU CAN, AS OFTEN AS YOU CAN.

Quit Tobacco Use

Smoking suppresses HDL production. When you are ready to quit, pick a date and create a quit plan. Remember to address not only the physical addiction but the psychological addiction as well. Have strategies in place for dealing with your triggers—stress, anger, anxiety, boredom, "the habit." Many of the reasons you reach for a cigarette are a normal part of life. Having an alternative for these triggers will enable you to quit for life!

Address Your Stress

During true fight or flight, we need extra fuel to mobilize the body and brain. This extra production of fuel leads the liver to produce increased amounts of LDL. Chronic, unmanaged stress means the liver is continually producing extra LDL. In addition, the stress response allows the body to hang onto fat (i.e., triglycerides), because the body thinks you are going to use it for fuel sooner rather than later. When this doesn't happen, you now have elevated triglycerides in the bloodstream and possibly a little extra unnecessary padding.

A physical outlet (EXERCISE!!) as well as a mental outlet for stress are both critical for health and wellness. Deep breathing, meditation, journaling, therapy—anything that helps get the thoughts out and quiets the mind will help shut off the stress response.

Sleep

It is not clearly understood how sleep deprivation affects cholesterol levels, but it is clear that it does. Women who consistently get fewer than six hours of sleep per night, may have low HDL and high triglyceride levels. Men are found to have higher LDL numbers. Of course, the other choices made regularly have a significant impact on these numbers. When you are sleep deprived, you may be making poor food choices and may not be exercising,

Identify your barriers to quality sleep—stress, interruptions, modern stimulants, nutrition, and exercise. Modify behaviors in these areas and you will probably notice an improvement in your sleep.

BMI

Dear Medical Community, PLEASE PLEASE PLEASE stop promoting BMI as a measure of health or disease. BMI is strictly a height/weight ratio. Because it does not factor in muscle mass, bone density, or bone structure, in my opinion, it is not an accurate reflection of a healthy weight. I think we can all look in the mirror and know if we have some body fat to lose, so I encourage people to ignore BMI and pay attention to body fat percentage, waist circumference, and waist-hip ratio instead.

BODY FAT PERCENTAGE

If you know anything about muscle tissue, you know that it is very dense. It doesn't take up a lot of space, but in its compact form, it is quite heavy. Does anyone remember when Oprah wheeled out her wagon of fat? It was 67 pounds—representing the amount of weight she had lost. It was a rather large pile. Imagine if that were 67 pounds of brick. It would take up a fraction of the space, and yet, 67 pounds is 67 pounds. It brings to mind a trick my dad once played to see if I understood the concept of weight versus volume. What weighs more, a pound of lead or a pound of feathers? As a kid, I thought a pound of feathers must weigh less—they are so light and fluffy. Well, duh—a pound is a pound; the feathers just take up a LOT MORE SPACE.

If you are a slave to the number on the scale, I want nothing more than for you to stop obsessing about it! Break up with the idea that this number equals your worth. I promise you, it doesn't! In the next chapter I will tell you more about my experience with allowing the "number" to dictate my life and how it all changed when I embraced the magic of muscle. If you truly want to lose body fat and prevent fat gain in the future, muscle is your ally. By the end of this book, I hope you will dedicate to building and maintaining your muscles, even though it may mean you don't love the number on the scale!

WAIST CIRCUMFERENCE AND WAIST-HIP RATIO

By now you have probably heard that belly fat increases your risk for heart disease. In fact, it increases your risk for EVERY disease. Ideally, your waist circumference, when measured at your belly button, is no greater than half your height in inches. For the mathematically challenged, if you are five feet, six inches tall, that equals sixty-six inches. Your waist circumference should be less that thirty-three inches. Anything greater than that and you may be at risk for heart disease, diabetes, cancer, etc.

What is it about belly fat that puts you at risk, rather than butt or thigh fat? Why is it so special? Well, a variety of reasons! Your organs are housed in your midsection, and a thin layer of fat surrounding them actually provides protection. Too much, however, will diminish the ability to deliver oxygen and nutrition via the bloodstream. Your heart will be forced to work harder to deliver the goods, but, ultimately, they will still be left with reduced resources, affecting optimal functioning.

Belly fat also produces inflammatory molecules. Chronic inflammation is at the root of every disease process, and anytime we injure ourselves in any way, inflammation kicks in to prevent further harm and start the healing process. You can think of excess belly fat as an injury simply because it triggers the inflammatory response.

Belly fat also produces estrogen. As previously mentioned, we all have estrogen and we all need estrogen—we just don't need our bellies to produce it. With estrogen production from the belly, we are at risk for being in a state of estrogen dominance (not balanced with progesterone), which will lead to many symptoms affecting physical and mental health.

Waist-Hip Ratio is another good measure of disease risk. Measure your hips at the widest part of your buttocks and divide your waist circumference measurement by your hip circumference measurement. For women a ratio >.85 and for men a ratio >.9 puts you in an elevated risk category.

OK, so we know belly fat is dangerous, but how do we make sure we keep the waist whittled? We do lots and lots of sit-ups and crunches and planks and fancy ab exercises with silly gadgets we buy from infomercials, right? HA! Errr, no. If that was all that was necessary (or even helpful), we would have no problems! Americans spend billions of dollars each year on magic machines that claim to give you a svelte, trim waist. Clearly, it is not that simple. The real answers are revealed throughout this book.

You maintain a healthy weight and achieve appropriate waist circumference through:

- proper nutrition

- regular, consistent, and varied exercise

- managing your stress in a healthy way

- getting quality sleep

- maintaining hormonal balance

Yup . . . it's called the healthy lifestyle! Believe me, I wish it were as easy as doing crunches and planks, but as you will soon learn, nothing is easy. If it sounds too good to be true, just ignore it!

Congratulations, you've just completed a crash course in basic human functioning. And I do mean BASIC! By no means should this information be used as a substitute for a conversation with your doctor. Hopefully, it has inspired you to learn more about how your body works and how some of your habits are impacting your health and disease risk. The rest of the book is full of valuable information to help improve your status, but for now, here are some things to consider:

1. Schedule an appointment for complete lab
    work including:
        a. blood pressure
        b. fasting glucose

    c. lipid profile

    d. full thyroid panel

    e. estrogen and testosterone
       (depending on age and health status).

2. Commit to a thorough understanding of any levels out of a healthy range.

3. Identify habits to modify to improve numbers.

4. Read the books recommended in this chapter.

FINAL THOUGHTS

Your health is your most valuable asset, but it can become the one most neglected. How much care goes toward your car, your home, or your retirement fund? Devoting time, energy, and possibly money to your health will save you time, energy, and money in the long run. In addition, the life you lead will be much more enjoyable and fulfilling if you are free of disease or are able to manage it to minimize disruptions in your life. Staying current with preventive care visits and age-related screenings will enable you to make changes to your lifestyle choices if necessary, and even if your health challenges are due to a genetic predisposition, your choices DO matter. I know you care about your health because you are reading this book. Knowledge is power, but you have to do something with that knowledge. Your personal wellness journey may be long and complicated or simple and straightforward. Regardless of where you are starting and how it will look, going on this journey is a huge step in the right direction. Committing to improving your habits and your health is a beautiful act of kindness, and many will thank you for it—your children, your significant other, your family members, and most important, your future self! You deserve to be a Better Being, and I am so happy you've chosen me to be a guide. The first part of this book has been informational, but it's about to get real, and raw, and a little bit wild. I know you're ready, so let's go do this!

Chapter Two

THE TRUTH ABOUT WEIGHT LOSS

PRESENTED WITH ONE OF THE following options, which would you choose?

A. Starting today, if you follow a certain diet and exercise plan, you can lose 8 pounds in the next month.

B. Starting today, using a different approach, you can be 6 pounds lighter one year from now.

Weigh (pun intended!) this choice carefully. What's it going to be? I suppose it's only fair if I clue you into the caveat.

If you go with option A, your 8 pounds, plus a few more will be back one year from now. You will have started this process several times over the course of the year, and now, one year later you are going to do it again, but try really hard this time. You will lose those same 8 pounds, and maybe a few of the extras that tagged along, but eventually they will all come back, and 3 or 4 more for good measure.

If you go with option B, those 6 pounds will never come back. In another year 6 more pounds will be gone for good, and every year following, pounds will disappear until you have reached a point that you'd like to maintain. Your life will not have been noticeably disrupted, and you still will have enjoyed things you love.

Have you changed your mind? Maybe you've already embraced the fact that slow and steady is the way to go, so option B was your pick. If you have yet to break up with the diet mentality of option A, I hope this chapter convinces you to reconsider!

There really is no magic to losing weight—just burn more calories than you consume. Although that is simple in theory, in reality, many challenges stand in the way. How often have you made the weight-loss resolution? Too many to count? Years ago, after giving up life as a gymnast, I got fat. Really FAT. Going from a rather small, compact gymnast to busting out of size 12 clothes was quite an accomplishment! It took about two years to reach this pinnacle, which I will tell you more about in Chapter Seven. I spent the next five years resolving to lose the weight. I was going to "be good" and try harder. I went on this magic diet and found that magic exercise program. I lost some of the weight for a period of time, but never all of it for good. Try as I might, nothing "worked." Well, of course it didn't, because I had not really committed to changing my lifestyle behaviors. I so yearned to see a result that when it didn't come as fast as I wanted or as much as I wanted, I gave up! I felt I worked hard and saw nothing, and it wasn't worth it—so I would swing entirely the other direction. After a few days or weeks of this, I would again become completely disgusted with myself and resolve to be better and try even harder. This all-or-nothing mindset was definitely not working out the way I wanted it to! I would do it ALL right for a little bit, then NOTHING right for a much longer bit, and there is no way this strategy was going to get me to where I wanted to be.

Does this sound familiar to you? If you have been down a similar road, and are perhaps still traveling down that road, here is my advice—change course!!! My breakthrough came when I stopped focusing on weight loss and, instead, focused on changing my lifestyle. I knew that if I consistently engaged in behaviors that would help me create a caloric deficit, I would lose weight. I eliminated the artificial deadlines I had constantly placed on myself—I need to lose 10 pounds by the end of the month, or I want to lose 20 pounds by summer. I know you have made similar goals and maybe that's what you had in mind when you picked up this book. How has it worked for you so far? In the past, if I had been successful in reaching my goal, I would celebrate—basically by ceasing all the actions that helped me lose weight in the first place. Or if I didn't reach my goal, the cycle of sabotage set in. Either way, I was going backward, the scale was going up and it seemed hopeless. What madness this is, and yet I know this is still the course for many people. We are SO fixated on an outcome, ideally with little to no effort, and we want it now—preferably yesterday if we're honest. This IS NOT REALITY! We all know weight loss is possible, but if you gain it back, WHO CARES if you once lost it?

This chapter will provide a preview of information that is detailed later. Since I can't possibly tackle every concept at once, you'll have to trust me when I tell you I will explain how each of these ideas impacts our ability or inability to achieve and maintain a healthy weight. Because knowledge without an actual strategy to implement that knowledge is rather useless, my focus for this chapter is to outline how to set yourself up for success.

STEP #1: NO MORE DIETING!

Please, I beg you, stop going on diets! If you go on a diet, you are going to go off the diet. You will see amazing results when you are on it. You will probably feel deprived and be angry and hungry and most likely malnourished. You may become obsessed with food and exercise and might not be a very pleasant person. This is no way to live, and at some point you will decide you can't keep it up. So you'll go off the diet and you know what happens. The weight comes back, twice as fast as it came off, and it brings a few extra friends to the party that never want to leave. Right now, this minute, you are going to pinky swear to me that you will never ever go on a diet again. Like, EVER. Never.

Critical to my success was to identify the situations in which I was making choices that were preventing me from losing weight. Through lots of reflection, hard conversations (with myself and others), and plenty of trial and error, I created strategies to handle those situations. Some solutions were obvious, some required help from others, and some came about when I learned more about nutrition and the human body. None of it was easy. Sometimes it wasn't fun. And it didn't happen overnight. It was (and still is) a process that I have to stay on top of by being thoughtful in my choices.

STEP #2: THROW AWAY THE SCALE

The biggest change I had to make was my mindset and thought processes regarding food and exercise. I used to contemplate these decisions based on how a particular choice was going to affect my weight. Everything, and I mean everything, was dictated by what the scale said or was going to say. I would weigh myself in the morning when I got up, then again after I exercised (before I drank water), and again later in the day, and another time before I went to bed. I'd weigh myself after I had a dinner out and after I hardly ate anything all day. The scale's readout dictated what happened next. If I was pleased with the number, I felt pretty good about myself and allowed myself to cheat—but just a little bit. If it was a bad number, I was angry and felt hopeless—what was the point of all my hard work and sacrifice? Sometimes I would dig deep and exercise a little more or skip breakfast the next day. If there was a *really* bad number on the scale, I usually decided it didn't matter; I didn't care if I were fat forever, so I might as well go eat some ice cream. I know some people reading this cannot relate on any level to this scenario, but I also know most can. No matter what number appeared, it did not help me lose weight! If you have allowed the scale to determine your worth, your emotions, and your actions, please ditch it! We will find other ways of measuring progress, but the scale is just not necessary and often not helpful.

STEP #3: DETERMINE YOUR WHY

The healthy choice is the hard choice. By the end of this book you will be so sick of me saying that, but I am going to continue to say it, because it's true. Every class I teach and every person I coach, inevitably says, "It's hard." Yes—if it wasn't hard, I wouldn't have written a book or even have a career. Nobody would need help figuring it out if it wasn't hard. You will have to make hard choices consistently and for a long period of time to achieve an outcome you say you want, and you'll have to have a really powerful reason to make those hard choices. When life takes over, and you don't feel like doing something you know you should, or you want to do something you know won't help you lose weight, you are going to have to convince yourself to make the hard choice. This is your WHY. Your personally meaningful reason for making the hard choice over and over and over again. We will visit this idea throughout the book because your self-talk directs your actions, but since this is the weight-loss chapter, you have to answer the question, "WHY do I want to lose weight?" It has to be SPECIFIC and PERSONAL and MEANINGFUL. To illustrate, I am going to share the story of a client I used to work with. We'll call her Sally.

Sally had come to me after hearing me speak at several of her company's wellness classes. She had struggled with her weight most of her life and decided she was truly ready to make changes. After getting to know a bit of her history I asked Sally why she wanted to lose weight. Her answers were typical: I want to be healthy; I want to have energy; I want to look better. I think everyone always wants to be healthy, have energy, and look their best, so I asked her if those had been reasons in the past for why she wanted to lose weight. Yes, of course! So clearly, they must not be good enough reasons. I asked her for more—a more powerful reason to get the weight off and keep it off for good. She talked about her family—husband and two tween-age kids. She said she wanted to be a good role model and be able to participate in activities. OK, now we were getting somewhere, but still, she had a husband and kids for a while, and so far it hadn't led to long-term weight loss. I asked her to dig deep for this one and when I saw her the next time she showed me a picture that had been taken the previous summer. It was her family on a roller coaster—sort of. The four seats were her husband, her son, her daughter, and an empty seat. She was not allowed on the ride because she could not fit in the seat. She said this picture was a metaphor for her life, depicting how much she had missed out on because of her weight. She said she no longer wanted to be the empty seat. Now THAT is SPECIFIC and PERSONAL and MEANINGFUL!

WHAT'S YOUR WHY?

STEP #4: CREATE YOUR VISION

We all have great intentions and know for the most part what we need to do, but then life gets in the way and we lose sight of what we say we want to achieve. I am a huge believer in the power of our senses—in this case, sight. If you cannot visualize what it is you are trying to achieve, the likelihood you will accomplish it is pretty slim. You may think this is just a bunch of voodoo and hocus-pocus, but it has been shown time and again that our thoughts dictate our actions. Typically, our thoughts are negative and focused on the past, which means we are going nowhere fast. To help redirect the thinking and the action, we need reminders of what we have decided is important to us. Our long-term goals get lost in the day-to-day mud that goes on inside our heads; as time passes the strength of our conviction to make changes and accomplish a goal starts to wane. It is the constant visual reminder that will keep your resolve strong, serving to motivate you to make those hard choices.

The homework from the introduction should have you well on your way to establishing your vision and, hopefully, your vision board. If you have not done that, here is another opportunity! It can look any way you want it to, but it should embody exactly what YOU want YOUR life to look like. Cut out pictures from magazines or print them from the internet. Use words and phrases that motivate and inspire you. Assemble it on poster board or a sheet of paper. Whatever shape it takes, include the behaviors that will be necessary to achieve the outcome. I like to focus on the positive—the actions I am going to take—but some people find motivation in negative reinforcement. You may want to make one side of your board positive and put pictures, words, and phrases of what you are trying to avoid on the other side. This board should be in plain sight. Save a picture of it on your phone so you can look at it throughout the day. These constant reminders of what you are trying to achieve, and what you need to do to get there, will begin to carve the neurological pathways that will allow you to TRULY believe you can accomplish this goal.

STEP #5: SAY IT OUT LOUD

If you stay silent about your goals, keeping the ideas safely tucked away in your head, that is probably where they will stay—in your head. These ideas will never lead to real change. It is easy to give into the doughnuts if nobody knows you are trying to not eat doughnuts! We all need accountability to keep us moving in the right direction, and this starts with sharing your intentions. When you say it out loud, use first-person, positive, forward-thinking terms. We will dive deep into self-talk in Chapter Six, but it is such a HUGE key to success that I will introduce it here.

I know you think you are really good at multitasking, but you cannot be positive and negative at the same time. Nobody can—just not possible! If we use negative words—"I *can't* eat that," "I'm *not supposed* to have that," "I *shouldn't* do this"—we are focusing on and giving energy to something we REALLY want but are trying to avoid. We feel like victims who are sacrificing so much, and it often makes us want it more. Instead, phrases such as "Not right now but maybe later" or "I would love to, but I am choosing this instead" give power, because YOU are in control. Follow me through this next scenario (perhaps you can relate).

If I go into the break room at work and I see leftover cake (AND I LOVE CAKE), I tell myself I can't have cake. I will start to feel angry and deprived that I can't have cake, especially because it seems everyone else can have cake. It's not fair, and I feel sorry for myself, then I decide—fuck it; I'm going to have cake anyway. Then I am going to spend a lot of time being mad at myself for eating the cake when I said I wasn't going to do it . . . and I'll probably eat more cake to make myself feel better. If, instead, I walk into the break room and see cake, and I say to myself, "Wow, that cake looks delicious . . . maybe I will have a piece later. First, I am going to go back to my desk and eat X (insert healthy, tasty snack)." After eating my snack, I recognize that I feel really good about myself for making the better choice. I feel empowered to know I can continue to make better choices that are going to help me reach my goals. Words create an energy, and the energy creates a feeling, and the feeling leads to actions.

The reality is you CAN have whatever you want. That's right—you can. But if you have whatever you want as often as you want, you most likely will not reach the outcome you want. It all comes down to choices, and it is up to you to decide which result of making this choice is more important—the short-term impact or the long-term outcome.

STEP #6: ENLIST SUPPORT

We all know change is hard, but it is even more difficult if we try to do it alone. We are pack animals, and members of our pack serve to provide support in a variety of ways. Somewhere along the way it became a sign of weakness to ask for help. That is ridiculous! If you are not good at something, how do you expect to improve without asking for help? I suppose you can struggle along doing it on your own, but that's an inefficient, frustrating strategy. Instead, surround yourself with likeminded people. Do you know someone who is already engaging in the behaviors you are trying to implement? Do you know someone who is trying to achieve a similar goal and likely needs to establish the same new habits you are trying to establish? These people can guide, inspire, and motivate you. They can also help keep you accountable. Perhaps you need further education or advice and the aid of a professional is required. Build your support team however it will best serve you, but in each case, you need to clearly articulate how each person can help. We all give and receive support in different ways, so spend some time thinking about what you need and who is best suited to provide it.

One of the biggest obstacles people face is a saboteur. We all have them, and they typically fall under one of these categories:

- someone who doesn't realize what you are trying to accomplish

- someone who has no idea why a particular challenge is difficult for you

- someone who actually doesn't want you to succeed

Sometimes the reason we don't declare our intentions is because we would then actually have to follow through. If you are truly ready for change, this is exactly why you say it out loud! Perhaps you fear being questioned or mocked, or you think you are the only one who struggles with this particular issue. One of the most frequent comments I receive from people who attend my classes is they appreciate how honest I am when I share my stories and the difficulties I had with my own choices. They never would have guessed, looking at me standing in front of them, that I have the same thoughts and experiences they have. Although we are all unique individuals, we really are much the same in many ways. There is strength and power in the shared experience, so I encourage you to open up and be OK acknowledging that there are certain things you are just not that good at.

I used to beat myself up when I could not stop at just one cookie or a little bit of ice cream. What is wrong with me? I am so weak and have no willpower! I was envious of those people who easily walked past a plate of brownies and didn't even take a look, while I was scheming about how to eat as many as I could with nobody noticing. I elevated, to an absurdly high level, the people who passed on seconds and even higher those who politely declined the firsts. They are so much better than me, and I wish I could be more like them! It all changed when I just finally admitted I am not good at not eating sweets that are offered to me and really terrible at saying no when they are sitting in front of my face. I am good at a lot of things—this just isn't one of them. It doesn't make me less of a person or anyone else better than me. It was uncomfortable to admit this not only to myself but also out loud to friends and family. What is so silly is, it's not like they didn't know—they could see it! There also were those who didn't understand. I can't tell you how many times I heard things like, "Only eat it if you are hungry" or "Just portion out a little bit each day," and my favorite—"Just don't eat it." Wow! What incredible suggestions—like I had never thought of that! Clearly, if something like overeating is not their issue, they are simply not going to understand how someone else struggles with it. Here's the thing: they don't have to understand your issue in order to be supportive of you. Hopefully, after a very open and honest conversation, one that may be difficult to have, they will decide to support you in whatever way you determine will be helpful.

The person who is intentionally sabotaging your efforts to change is the most difficult one to deal with. If they are choosing to not support you, even after a heartfelt discussion, it is often for one of these reasons:

- it is highlighting their own need for change that either they are not yet admitting or are not ready to commit to.

- their motives relate to their insecurities

- they may just be assholes

"That's your problem, not mine" is a statement you are likely to hear. Ultimately, this is true and you need to make some choices: A—remove yourself from the environment. B—remove the saboteur from the environment. C—put a solid strategy in place, including your WHY and what you are going to do instead when the cookies come calling.

STEP #7: IDENTIFY YOUR OBSTACLES

Cliché alert—the path to success is paved with good intentions. I love clichés because they are TRUE! We all face obstacles; in fact, I think life is a series of obstacles, and if we don't have ways of getting around them, it will be a frustrating and unfulfilling life. A Better Being is not willing to accept that and will figure out ways of dealing with the things that are limiting growth and success. I just covered at length a common one—the saboteur. Awareness is key, so take time to identify what people, places, things, or situations might prevent you from participating in the behaviors necessary to reach your goal. These are your obstacles to success. The great news is there is an answer for everything (and I probably have it—just ask my parents). Some are easy to deal with, others require major decisions, but ALL are about choice.

Whether it is a tiny little bump or a seemingly insurmountable mountain, if you fail to have a system in place to deal with the obstacle, when you come upon it, you will turn around. Start with the easy ones to clear your path as much as you can as soon as you can. Reflect upon a time when you headed down this road before—what allowed you to be successful and what prevented it? It is quite likely you will be faced with these same challenges. Think through the strategy that will set you up for success. Write it down, use any tool to remind you, and start implementing it.

STEP #8: KEEP TRACK TO STAY ON TRACK

It is so easy to be a little off when we try to remember what we ate, how much we ate, when we last worked out, etc. We often underestimate what goes on and overestimate how much we move our bodies, which is not going to help the weight loss cause! I don't think you need to track forever, but I suggest you track for now. Measure your food and use an app (MyFitnessPal, Daily Burn, LoseIt!) or a good old-fashioned pencil-and-paper journal. Get an activity tracker (Fitbit, Garmin Connect, or my personal favorite, Misfit). You have to establish baseline behaviors before you know where you should focus your efforts. Once you have the baseline, look for opportunities for change and go about setting the SMART goals to facilitate those changes.

Specific—state exactly what are you trying to achieve
Measure it—how you will keep track
Actions—actions that need to happen for this outcome to be achieved
Realistic—be sure what you are proposing to do is realistic in your current life
Time to check in—your plan to stay accountable

I know SMART goals are annoying and tedious to write, but they are also very effective. Change does not come about by hoping or wishing or trying; it comes about by DOING. I learned this at a young age. I would often whine to my coach, "I'm trying!" His response was to stop trying and start doing. It may sound a bit harsh, but it's true. You have to be a doer if you want anything to happen.

OK, you are ready to start doing, but what exactly is necessary to lose weight? Once you have created a deficit of 3,500 calories, you will have lost 1 pound of body fat. That means you have to burn 3,500 more calories than you put in your body. For those of you who have tracked intake and output, you know this is a GIGANTIC number. It is calories in-calories out, which looks easy on paper but is a bit more complicated in real life. The three keys to creating that deficit for lasting results are: calorie intake modification, increased energy output, and hormonal balance.

CALORIE INTAKE MODIFICATION

I am never going to call it "going on a diet," because that implies that it is for a fixed amount of time. Lasting results come from making lifelong changes. Most likely you will need to modify what is going in—maybe the amount of food, the types of foods, or how and when you are eating your food. You see, the type of calories that go in, the way they go in, and when they go in affect how (if at all) they go out! Let's see if I can make sense of this for you.

You Need to Eat!

One of the biggest mistakes people make when they are trying to lose weight is cutting too many calories. I know it seems like it should work—and it may for a while—but once you start eating again, you will regain the weight. Here's why: Back in the day the only reason you didn't eat was because there was no food to eat. In order to survive the food shortage, the body conserves energy (does not burn calories) and releases cortisol. The release of cortisol directs fat storage around your belly to protect your organs while you are losing weight during the food shortage. When you can no longer exist on the meager number of calories the environment is providing you (in the case of our ancestors, food scarcity; in the case of us, the newest diet), you will eat more—sometimes A LOT more. The body responds with a "WOOT-WOOT—the famine is over, we are in feasting mode!" And just to make sure you survive the next famine, you will hang onto a little more than you had before.

Resting metabolic rate (RMR), also known as Resting Energy Expenditure (REE), is the number of calories you need to simply exist. If you were to lie in bed all day and do nothing, your body would burn a certain number of calories for basic functioning—for your heart to beat, lungs to contract, cells to turn over, etc. If you are doing more than lying still for 24 hours, you need to eat a bit more than your RMR number of calories. If you eat less, you have indicated that there is a food shortage and your body slows down every process—affecting the calories out part of the equation. If weight loss is your goal, you should never, ever, ever eat fewer than your RMR number of calories. A calculator will make it easy by asking for your height, weight, age, and gender, but here are the longhand formulas for men and women using the Mifflin-St. Jeor equation.

RMR FORMULA

Men: Resting metabolic rate = (10 x W) + (6.25 x H) - (5 x A) + 5

Women: Resting metabolic rate = (10 x W) + (6.25 x H) - (5 x A) - 161

W = weight in pounds   H = height in inches   A = age in years

Using longhand math, let's walk through the calculation for the following metrics:

Gender: Female
Height: 5'6"= 66"
Weight: 155 lbs
Age: 45

(10 x 155) + (6.25 x 66) - (5 x 45) -161
(1,550) + (412.5) - (225) - 161= 1,576.5

RESTING METABOLIC RATE = 1,576.5

This formula will give a pretty good estimate of what your RMR is, but it cannot be exact. Percentage of muscle mass, bone structure, and hormones also influence your RMR, but it is nearly impossible to measure those with accuracy and put it into a neat formula.

You should never eat fewer than your RMR number of calories, but if you are aiming to lose weight, you still need to create a deficit of input versus output. So how many calories should you be eating? It depends on many factors and estimating your total daily energy expenditure is a good starting point. TDEE is the number of calories you burn on any given day. For most people, no two days are exactly the same. There are days I am driving all over town to train clients and teach onsite wellness classes. When it's all added up, I could be sitting in the car for up to six hours. There are other days I stay home and teach webinars back-to-back, clean my house, and go up and down the levels of my building. The energy expenditure of those two days is very different, because standing and moving around expend much more energy than sitting. The day I climb a fourteener (a mountain of at least 14,000 feet) versus the day I lie on the couch and watch football are VERY different levels of output. Think about how you spend your days—how much variance is there in the amount of and intensity of the movement? When calculating TDEE, take a few scenarios that reflect a variety of ways you spend your days. This will illustrate how much impact movement has on your caloric expenditure. You can get a rough estimate of TDEE by using a calculator that asks you to input exactly how you are spending every minute of your day.

As stated above, the types of calories that go in, the way they go in, and when they go in also affect how the body burns those calories. I have not yet even adjusted for muscle mass and hormone levels/balance. It's complicated, right?

Health-calc.com is a great website that has a variety of calculators to help you figure out these things. Set aside some time to devote to learning how to navigate the site. Once you enter in all your stats, it will calculate approximately how many calories you burn in a day. Based on that, you can start modifying intake and increasing output. Remember, the information you get out is only as good as the information you put in. We definitely overestimate how much we are moving our bodies as well as the intensity of the movement, so be very thoughtful and as precise as possible when inputting your data.

Calories Going In

Now that you have an idea of how many calories you burn a day, and you know you need to eat the minimum (RMR), you can decide how to create your deficit. Nutrition modification will most likely be required, and the next chapter covers nutrition in depth. I am going to give it to you here in a nutshell to get your head wrapped around a few critical concepts.

1. **PFF is your BFF.**
   Yes, you get to embrace a new best friend—the combination of protein, fat, and fiber. It is going to be your BFF for so many reasons, but it aids in weight loss in a few ways: it keeps your blood sugar steady, reduces hunger, and helps signal you are full. More in Chapter Three, but for now start paying attention to your food combinations. Every time you eat, there should be protein, fat, and fiber.

2. **Eat every 2–4 hours.**
   Again, it's about steady blood sugar. That really is the goal from the time you get up to the time you go to bed. As you use your fuel throughout the day, you need to refuel. If you go too long without eating, the body will start to prepare for the famine!

3. **Eat early and often.**
   Eat most of your calories often and early in the day; eat fewer as you get closer to bedtime. We need fuel while we are up and functioning, not when we are about to lie down to go to sleep.

4. **Get real with your food.**
   Put mostly REAL, high-quality WHOLE foods in your body and minimize the things that come in a carton, wrapper, bag, or box, or from a restaurant.

5. **Engage in mindful eating.**
   Make yourself WAITE—Why am I tempted to eat? If it is

for any reason other than physical nourishment, it better be worth it!

MAXIMIZING CALORIC EXPENDITURE

Now that you have a sense of how the calories going in impact how they go out, let's look at how our movement affects the process. Calories are the form of energy the body uses to accomplish movement. The more you move and the higher the degree of intensity, the more energy is expended. Chapter Four details all components of fitness, but let's explore a few key concepts here to get you started.

Activity

All movement can contribute to creating your caloric deficit. Activity is simply the movement required to get through your day. The minimum amount a human body desires is 10,000 steps. There is no magic to this number, but it is close to what our prehistoric ancestors did in the natural course of a day. If you have a sedentary job, you have a big hurdle to jump. Most likely you are in the 2,500-3,500 range of steps without adding in deliberate movement. Your first goal is to become human! You have to figure out how to get more movement in your day. In addition, you need get up every hour to keep metabolism (the rate at which the body burns calories) up and running. Back in the day the only reason you were immobile for an extended period of time was because you were sick, injured, or dying. To prolong life, the body slows down and conserves energy. Nowadays, you are not sick, injured, or dying— you are just sitting. Maybe you are working or driving a vehicle or watching TV, but you are not physically doing anything. Your goal is to create a caloric deficit—to maximize the calories out part of the equation, and every little thing counts. If you can stand instead of sit, stand. If you can move around instead of standing still, move around. If you can move around at a higher level of intensity, do it. Once you pass on a chance to burn calories, you don't get it back!

Exercise

All components of exercise are important, but for weight loss, regular cardiovascular activity AND strength training are critical.

When engaging in cardiovascular activity, the harder you work the more calories you burn, and to even be considered exercise you need to work in your target heart rate zone. There are a few formulas for calculating THRZ, but my preferred one is the Karvonen Formula. This one takes into consideration your resting heart rate, which makes it a more accurate calculation. To determine resting heart rate, you need to check it right upon waking, ideally before you even sit up. If your activity tracker has a heart rate feature, check the reading when you wake up. Otherwise, have a stopwatch positioned by your bed and take a 30-second heart rate count. Multiply by 2 to determine your beats per minute and enter this number into the formula. It is an extremely long and complicated formula, but there are plenty of websites that will let you plug your number in and give you your target heart rate zone. A less accurate but very easy calculation is:

220−age = Max Heart Rate

65%–85% of Max Heart Rate = Target Heart Rate Zone

Someone age 45 would have a Max Heart Rate of
175 beats per minute and a

Target Heart Rate Zone of 114 to 149 beats per minute.

Often the question is "How much do I have to do?"
Keep in mind the goal is to create a caloric deficit and the more you move the more you burn. My advice is:

DO AS MUCH AS YOU CAN, AS HARD AS YOU CAN, AS OFTEN AS YOU CAN!

As important, if not more, is strength training. This is often neglected for a variety of reasons. Some people are still under the impression that because you burn more calories during a cardio workout than a strength training workout, this is not an effective use of time. I was one of these people back in the early days of my weight-loss efforts. I was the cardio queen—I walked everywhere whenever I could, I did sixty to ninety minutes of cardio exercise five or six days a week, and often threw in an extra aerobics class or bike ride if I had the time. The trainer at the gym would encourage me to lift weights, and I dabbled in it a bit, but my main focus was cardio. Gotta burn calories, gotta sweat, gotta keep moving! I lifted weights a bit as a gymnast for our conditioning before the season started, but that was to be strong. I didn't connect it with how it impacts weight loss. While in graduate school learning more about exercise physiology, I decided to give it a go and see for myself what all the fuss was about. I committed to strength training, I mean really strength training, for three months. Turns out muscle is magical! The scale didn't actually move that much, but I was smaller—by about three sizes. As we discussed earlier, muscle is very dense. It doesn't take up much space, but for that space, it weighs a lot, which is yet another reason to ditch the scale. I don't know about you, but I would much prefer a higher number on the scale with a lower number on my pants tag than the other way around.

I will detail more about the magic of muscle in Chapter Four, but trust me when I say that muscle is your ally if you are trying to lose body fat! Although you may not burn as many calories during the workout, muscle itself is metabolically active, meaning it requires calories just to exist. Muscle burns calories 24-7 unlike fat, which sits around and doesn't do much. If maximizing caloric output is the goal, having muscle working for you seems like a sound strategy!

Consistency is super important because muscles begin to decondition approximately 72 hours after you've used them. Work each muscle group 2–3 times a week. You also need to lift weight that is heavy enough to challenge your muscles to do more than they want to. This is how you build muscle mass, which boosts your metabolism. I will expand on these tips in Chapter Four but for now, just start lifting something. The more muscle you have the higher your resting metabolic rate will be so . . .

HUSTLE, HUSTLE BUILD THAT MUSCLE!

Hormonal Balance

You learned in Chapter One that hormones rule your world, and your ability or inability to lose weight is no exception. Although there are many factors that influence our weight, I will outline a few of the major players and how our habits may throw them out of balance.

Insulin

Refresher on the function of insulin: When we eat food that contains carbohydrates, it gets broken down into glucose. Glucose in the bloodstream triggers the release of insulin from the pancreas. Insulin is the key to unlocking the cells, which open up and let the glucose in to be used as fuel. If we eat a lot of food all at once, previously known as a feast, the body will make sure to store some for later use. Your storage builds up on the thighs, hips, and buttocks, and in the abdominal area, just waiting to be tapped into. This will come in handy when we face a famine, except that is unlikely to happen for most of us!

Prevent the overproduction of insulin by keeping blood sugar steady. Eat PFF every 2–4 hours, consume most calories early and often, and stay in the calorie budget appropriate for your needs and goals.

Ghrelin and Leptin

Do you think hunger hormones play a role in weight loss or

gain? Um, duh. It's really hard to minimize what is going in if you are hungry all the time and never truly satiated. Ghrelin is produced in the lining of your stomach and is released to tell you to eat so you don't die of starvation or malnourishment. Leptin is produced and released from your fat cells to tell you to stop eating so you don't overdo it and end up with too much storage. The pattern of eating—whether it is not enough or not frequently enough—will trigger the release of ghrelin. Sleep deprivation, chronic stress, and a low-functioning thyroid can all skew the production, leading to higher levels of ghrelin and lower levels of leptin. When these are out of balance or the messages they are sending are no longer recognized, it can compound the struggles with a weight-loss effort.

To keep ghrelin in check you need to fuel properly. Refer back to the "Calories Going In" section in this chapter for details. Fiber, in particular, is going to be helpful in shutting off the ghrelin signal. Fiber acts as a sponge, and as it travels through the digestive system, it absorbs water. By the time it has reached the stomach, the quantity of food has grown tremendously in volume, taking up plenty of space. When you are full of healthy food, there is little room for much else. In addition, as the stomach lining stretches, ghrelin production shuts down—basically your stomach stops screaming at you because the "I'm HUNGRY" message is no longer being sent.

Getting 7–9 hours of quality sleep and practicing healthy stress management are also critical for healthy ghrelin and leptin levels. There will be much more on those conepts in Chapters Six and Eight.

Leptin is more responsible for the satiety signal, and trouble arises when you build up leptin resistance—you are no longer receptive to the message that you are satisfied. It works much the same as insulin resistance, where your body stops responding to the message from insulin for cells to open up and let the glucose in. In fact, research is showing that insulin resistance and leptin resistance are somewhat intertwined. Avoid leptin resistance by properly nourishing yourself (again—refer to the "Calories Going In" section). If you are diabetic or pre-diabetic, you should consider limiting the intake of fructose, the type of sugar found in fruit, to no more than 20g per day. Everyone should stay away from high-fructose corn syrup (HFCC), as this sweetener has the most dramatic impact on blood sugar spikes, which we want to avoid at all costs!

Cortisol

I have mentioned several times that cortisol is released anytime there is a threat to the body—whether real or perceived. When cortisol is out of balance, many things are out of balance. Depending on the nature of the threat it may direct the body to conserve energy or store fat around the belly. Keep cortisol in check by maintaining steady blood sugar, minimizing caffeine and alcohol consumption, getting regular quality sleep, and minimizing your fight-or-flight response. MUCH more on that will be discussed in Chapter Six.

TSH

Thyroid-stimulating hormone is the granddaddy of them all, affecting every process in the human body. It may affect your weight because low-functioning thyroid can result in fatigue, joint and muscle pain, and a slow metabolism. It can also trigger sugar cravings. Low-functioning thyroid affects millions and millions of people, many of whom will go undiagnosed or inadequately treated. An important concept to embrace is the difference between "normal" and "optimal." If you have had your thyroid tested and your doctor said you are normal . . . push back! The reference range is as wide as the ocean and how you feel at the low end of normal versus the high end of normal is vastly different.

I tested in the mid-range of "normal" but wanted to see

what life was like at the optimal level. With the help of my for-ward-thinking, patient-centered doctor, I began a very low dose of desiccated (T4/T3 combo) thyroid medicine. I did not have many of the serious symptoms of low-functioning thyroid, but I have absolutely seen significant changes, most notably in my sugar cravings, hunger level, and chronic joint pain. My hair and nails are growing faster than ever, and it's nice not to have icy hands and feet. At this point in my life my weight is not a serious concern, but I have enjoyed the benefit of losing a few pounds. It does make me wonder how much easier my weight-loss effort might have been if back in my twenties, I had known what I know now. At that time, I did have my thyroid levels tested and was told I was "normal." I suspect then I was at the low end of the range and believe a low dose of the right medicine would have dramatically changed the duration of my journey.

Estrogen, Progesterone, and Testosterone

The sex hormones play critical roles in our weight, and bal-anced, optimal levels keep us healthy. I have heard countless times, "It's not fair; my husband loses weight so much easier than I do." That's right, ladies, it's not fair, but it is reality! Of course, men have more testosterone than women—MUCH more—and due to all that testosterone, they are able to build and maintain lean muscle mass. We know muscle burns calories all the time and the more you have the more you burn. Women have testos-terone as well, and even though it is only about 10 percent of the amount found in men, it is extremely critical. Having optimal tes-tosterone levels can result in more energy and more muscle mass, both of which can aid in weight loss. There is a natural decline in testosterone production (and all sex hormones) as we age, but there are also some lifestyle habits that could contribute to low levels. What's really important is how much free testosterone is available for the body to use. Each hormone has a binding globu-lin, and production of the sex-hormone-binding globulin (SHBG) can be increased with lack of exercise, alcohol consumption, obesity, and certain medications. Higher levels of SHBG will result in lower levels of free testosterone, because the testosterone that is produced is "bound up." Lifestyle changes must be included in any type of protocol for maximum results.

Estrogen and progesterone have direct and indirect impacts on our weight. It is much too complicated for me to get into all the roles they play, so I am going to keep it simple. When we are YBI (young, beautiful, invincible), estrogen and progesterone are equal partners, playing nicely with each other. As we go through the aging process and enter the phase of perimenopause, there is a dramatic plummet in progesterone production. The result is estrogen dominance. Estrogen dominance leads to all kinds of things going horribly wrong and is related to many physical and mental health issues including cancer, heart disease, autoimmune conditions, migraines, and depression, just to name a few. Water retention and weight gain are also consequences of estrogen dominance.

Both men and women can find themselves in a state of estrogen dominance because many of our lifestyle choices lead to this condition. Obesity (particularly belly fat), a low-fiber diet, hormones, and antibiotics in the food supply, and a lack of exercise are just a few ways the body ends up producing too much estrogen. Chronic stress and adrenal fatigue can lead to low progesterone production.

Ideally, our sex hormones, as well as all of our hormones, are at optimal and balanced levels. I encourage people to get their levels tested then determine the best course of action. But before taking any action, I again highly recommend these books: *Stop the Thyroid Madness* by Janie A. Bowthorpe, M.Ed. and *How to Achieve Healthy Aging* by Dr. Neal Rouzier for explanations about many important hormones that everyone can understand. Hormone replacement is not a decision to enter into lightly or without fully understanding the process, so please be an informed participant in your own health. Do your homework and your research then get ready for a possibly arduous and frustrating process before you finally have the answers you are looking for. It won't be fun, but it will be well worth the effort in the long run!

There you have it—The Truth About Weight Loss! I know it is probably not the answers you were looking for, but by now you can probably tell I pull no punches. Reality is often hard work and many times not fun, but living with delusions of a quick fix is not any fun either. If you are ready to stop dieting and change your lifestyle for good, here are some things to consider:

1. Go through Steps #1–#8 to create a solid strategy for your weight-loss journey.

2. Make a list of healthy foods you like.

3. Track intake for one week to get a baseline of habits.

4. Invest in an activity tracker.

5. Calculate your RMR and your THRZ.

FINAL THOUGHTS

Your outcome will be a product of all the behaviors you engage in consistently over time. Imagine if five years ago you had gradually changed habits that resulted in just a pound or two of weight loss each month. See yourself a year from now or five years from now. What do you look like? How do you feel? What are you doing? Successfully losing weight is like anything else, and if you maximize the opportunities to create a caloric deficit, and you do that consistently and for an extended period of time, YOU WILL LOSE WEIGHT. There is not one choice that is going to make you skinny or one choice that will leave you fat. If you did something that you weren't intending, and it is getting you further away from your goal, it's OK! It is not the end of the world if you ate a cookie—or ten cookies. You are not a failure if you only worked out twice and you planned on four times. In life we either win or we learn, and it is only failure if you choose not to learn from the experience. The journey of a Better Being has many twists and turns and ups and downs. Weight loss will most likely require more effort than you think it should and take longer than you want it to, but the important thing is to stay headed in the right direction and make progress! Identify the challenges, celebrate the successes, and keep on going!

Chapter Three

WHAT AM I
SUPPOSED TO EAT?

HOW MANY TIMES HAVE YOU asked yourself that question? Nutrition plays a key role in our health, but confusion is found around every corner, and what's good for us today is going to kill us tomorrow. Food is complex chemistry and the human body is complex chemistry. When you mix two sets of complex chemicals, the reactions can vary dramatically. What is "healthy" for one person is not necessarily a good choice for someone else. As I outlined in the previous chapter, after I quit gymnastics, I got fat. It's not rocket science why that happened—I was eating too many things that had too many calories and not enough things that gave my body high-quality nutrients. In many of the cases, I thought I was making good choices, only to later learn that I was actually setting myself up for giving into the food I said I wasn't going to eat. I often found myself asking what was wrong with me and eventually realized I just didn't understand complex chemistry. Figuring out what I am supposed to eat was, and has continued to be, a journey all its own. I have made some incredible discoveries along the way that truly have changed my life and the lives of many people who have embraced and implemented the concepts I am going to outline for you. A basic understanding of nutrition is helpful, so we'll start with Nutrition 101.

CARBS, PROTEIN, AND FAT—THE MACROS

Thanks to CrossFit and MyFitnessPal, "macros" is the hot term right now. Carbohydrates, protein, and fat are the macro (big) nutrients your body uses. These are the ones that provide energy in the form of calories. Each macronutrient comes in a variety of forms. Some taste delicious and provide high-quality nutrition and some taste more delicious and provide us pleasure. We also need the micronutrients—vitamins, minerals, and water. For ideal functioning each macronutrient would like to play with the others in a particular ratio. Each micronutrient also has a specific ideal ratio with its pals for the body to thrive. Abundance or deficiencies of any of the macros or micros will lead to imbalance, which eventually leads to compromised physical or mental well-being.

Carbohydrates

Contrary to some popular diets, I believe we need to consume all of the macronutrients, but most of us can use an adjustment when it comes to certain ones. In my experience, both personally and professionally, the typical American consumes way too many carbohydrates. It's easy to do because they are everywhere, in our healthy foods and our pleasure foods, and they are relatively cheap and convenient.

Not only are carbohydrates NOT the enemy, but they are critical for energy and brain function! They are also your only source of fiber. What typically comes to mind when someone mentions carbs are visions of fresh warm bread, a plate of pasta, or a hearty mound of mashed potatoes. True, these are foods made up primarily of carbohydrates, but there are so many more. If it is a plant or comes from a plant, or the food has a naturally occurring sugar, it is a source of carbohydrates. Fruits, vegetables, whole grains, beans, seeds, nuts, and dairy foods are all made up of carbohydrates.

When you put food in, the body is going to work hard to break it down into its raw materials. Carbohydrates are made up of some combination of fiber, starch, and a form of sugar specific to each type of food. Dairy foods have no starch or fiber, so the lactose (the form of sugar in dairy) gets broken down to glucose. Fruit has fructose and fiber, so in the body we end up with glucose and fiber. Beans have oligosaccharides, starch, and fiber, leaving us with glucose, starch, and fiber. You see a theme here? The SUGAR form found in the food gets converted into GLUCOSE in the body. Glucose is the form of sugar the human body uses for fuel. We need glucose; we just tend to get too much of it, and if we are not eating it with protein and fat, it could cause some problems. In Chapter Two I introduced PFF as your BFF, and you learned one of the primary reasons you will never eat a carbohydrate by itself is because you know this will lead to a spike in blood sugar followed by a crash.

Roughly 40–50 percent of your overall calories should come from carbs—mostly vegetables, a bit of fruit, some beans, seeds, and nuts, and perhaps some whole grains. Because the color of the fruit or vegetable indicates what nutrients it offers, pile your cart with a rainbow of colors. These will give you a nice dose of disease-fighting vitamins and antioxidants—like medicine to suppress and reverse the disease process and help your body to heal.

Minimize or avoid the refined and processed carbohydrates. These include white bread, pasta, tortillas, and rice, as well as juice and sweetened drinks. Of course, "treats" also fall into this category—baked goods, chips, ice cream, candy, etc. In the case of refined grains, the mill has done the work your body is supposed to do. It has stripped the grain of the protein and fiber, leaving just a simple sugar for your body to deal with. It is TOO easy to break down a simple sugar, which causes the spike that leads to the crash. Remember, steady blood sugar is one of the keys to optimal health, and consuming a simple sugar without protein and fat is the enemy of steady blood sugar.

Fiber

One of the most important reasons to consume high-quality sources of carbohydrates is to ensure we take in an adequate amount of fiber. The body cannot digest fiber, which comes in many forms but falls into two categories—soluble and insoluble. Soluble fiber dissolves in water and serves as "food" for our good gut bacteria. Insoluble fiber does not dissolve in water and helps keep your digestive system and colon happy. Since it cannot be digested, it spends a long time in the bloodstream, where the body is attempting to break it down. This helps keep our blood sugar steady—preventing those spikes and crashes. In addition, fiber helps keep us full. It acts as a sponge, absorbing water and expanding in the stomach. It literally takes up space, which means there is no room for other things! As the stomach expands with the volume of food, it stretches the stomach lining, which shuts off the production of ghrelin (your hunger hormone). Just another reason PFF is your BFF! To get a wide variety of the many different types of fiber, eat whole plant foods! If it is a plant or comes from a plant, it will have fiber. Aim for 14 grams of fiber for every 100 pounds of your body weight. A 200-pound person would want a minimum of 28 grams of fiber each day. Make sure you are taking in plenty of water to keep it all moving along to avoid discomfort of another kind!

Protein

Cellular growth, brain development, and muscle formation are just a few of the important roles requiring protein. It is also needed for cell structure and for function and regulation of tissues and organs. Proteins form in the body by taking a variety of amino acids, linking them together to form peptide chains that assemble in a variety of combinations to perform different duties. Acting as messengers (hormones), enzymes (lactase), and transporters (ferritin) are just a few examples of the roles proteins play. In order for it to work, we must consume foods that provide amino acids the body can't produce. Chicken, eggs, red meat, dairy, and nuts are foods we think of as protein. But these are simply foods that have amino acids our bodies can use to produce the peptide chains (i.e., proteins).

Including a wide variety of food sources is always my recommendation. Many people think they consume enough protein, but in reality, they usually fall well short. The body can produce many of its own amino acids, but there are nine that it cannot make. We call them essential amino acids. It is ESSENTIAL we eat foods that have them or the peptide chains they are part of cannot be formed, and without those peptide chains, their duties cannot be performed. Not all protein sources are created equally! Animal sources are complete proteins, meaning they contain all essential amino acids. The plant-based proteins lack one or more of the essential amino acids, making them incomplete. However, you can combine two incompletes to form a complete protein. Having some type of whole grain with a bean or nut would constitute a complete protein.

Optimally, 25–30 percent of your caloric intake should come from protein. One of the main challenges in accomplishing this is many foods we eat do not have that much protein. Here are some examples:

1 egg = 7-9 grams

½ cup beans = 9-11 grams

¼ cup nuts = 8-10 grams

1 ounce cheese = 8-10 grams

1 cup Greek yogurt (depending on the brand) = 16–23 grams

3 ounces chicken = 23 grams

To illustrate why it is so difficult to achieve adequate protein intake, let's take the example of a person taking in 2,000 calories/day, with 30 percent of those calories coming from protein.

2,000 cal x 30% = 600 calories from protein

Protein has 4 cal/gram

600/4 = 150 grams of protein

It would require a tremendous amount of nuts, cheese, eggs, and beans to get close to 150 grams of protein. However, because those foods come with other sources of calories, it will be nearly impossible to stay on a calorie budget that is appropriate for your needs and goals and get the protein you need without going over the percent of those calories coming from carbohydrates and possibly fat.

If you are vegetarian or vegan, it is nearly impossible to get adequate protein in your diet. Most people, even those who do consume meat, would benefit from a high-quality protein powder as part of their daily diet. I go two ways with protein powder, and it comes down to what it is giving me and what it is costing me.

If I am going to make a smoothie with a liquid base of unsweetened almond or coconut milk and delicious ingredients like greens, berries, nut butter, or coconut oil, I will opt for a very clean, organic whey protein with no sweeteners and nothing artificial, which on its own tastes disgusting. What it is giving me is high-quality protein with no junk added. What does it cost me? I have to make a smoothie—and clean the blender.

If I need something quick that I will drink, it needs to taste delicious. In that case I opt for a low-sugar (typically stevia as the sweetener), chocolate-flavored whey protein. I combine ½ cup unsweetened coconut milk with 1½ cups of water, add my protein powder, and shake, shake, shake. A dash of cinnamon is fun and sometimes I add a splash of leftover coffee. What does this give me? A delicious drink I have on the go that takes minimal time and effort to prepare—and nothing but a simple bottle to clean. What it costs me is most likely introducing some artificial ingredients into my body. Although that is not ideal, I know that the alternative of not having a protein shake will most likely be some version of carbohydrate and probably not a very healthy one!

Fat

Let's talk about fat, baby. Let's talk about it, you and me. Let's talk about all the good things and the bad things that we eat. Let's talk about fat! Yes, I just added a little Salt-N-Pepa to the discussion. But I do LOVE talking about fat. Poor thing is so misunderstood and feared and even hated by some. I used to fear and hate it too, because I learned it was the devil! In the '80s and '90s we were told fat is the enemy that is going to kill us all. If we eat fat, we will get fat, then heart disease, then die. So, I, along with much of America, embraced the fat-free craze. I made "healthy" choices like fat-free yogurt, cereal, skim milk, bagels with fat-free cream cheese, and lots of fruit—basically anything that didn't have fat. Frozen yogurt and SnackWells cookies and fat-free cereal bars were staples in my daily diet. As long as I didn't eat fat, I was going to be A-OK! My love for peanut butter made it tricky to not eat fat, so I got used to the reduced-fat version. It was pretty gross but worth the sacrifice, because it would save me from getting fat and dying. I stopped eating eggs and butter and substituted red meat with chicken. Being from Wisconsin and of Dutch heritage, cutting out cheese was a challenge, but, hey, if it means I won't get fat, I'll do it!

Imagine my shock, dismay, and sense of defeat when I got fat. How could this be? I did everything they told me to do. I was exercising like I should, and I was eating a basically fat-free diet, so how could I be getting fat? OK, I suppose the cookies and cake and ice cream that I couldn't seem to say no to had something to do with it. But, I swear, I tried really hard not to eat those things. I would start out each morning "being good." I dutifully ate my half a plain bagel, fat-free yogurt, and a banana, always starting out the day so determined not to have any sweets, but within a few hours it was useless. I caved, I succumbed, and I found my way to the sugar. Good god what is wrong with me? Why do I have NO willpower? Why can't I just stay away from these things? The mental lashings I inflicted were brutal. Usually I got to the point where I decided I was a loser and might as well just eat what I wanted. If I had known then what I know now, how different my life might have been.

I now know not only is fat NOT THE DEVIL, but it is my ANGEL, sent from food heaven to correct all the wrongs. If you still fear fat, think it will make you fat and give you heart disease, I plan to change your mind. If you are not eating enough fat, you are most likely eating too many carbohydrates. You see, it is not simply the foods you are eating that matter, it is the ratio of the nutrients you are taking in. Ideal ratio for steady blood sugar is:

40% of the calories come from carbs

30% of the calories come from protein

30% of the calories come from fat

To calculate the percentages every time you eat is way too much math for an individual (although I have had a woman in my classes who did just that for all of her PFF combinations!). If at the very least you get on the PFF is your BFF bandwagon, you will be well on your way. I think it would be beneficial to use a tracker that calculates the percentages to help identify where you might be out of balance. You may find you are eating a lot of healthy foods, but it is too much of some things and not enough of others. Generally, it is too many calories from carbohydrates and not enough calories from protein and fat. That is when you are being "good." When you are not being good, it is too many carbs, not enough protein, and too much fat—because it is also too many calories!

Let's get into the nitty-gritty of good fats and bad fats. It gets complicated, but I warned you that food is complex chemistry. In the effort to simplify the message, sometimes the message gets completely distorted. Such is the case with the good fat vs. bad fat debate. You may have heard or read things along these lines:

Saturated fats are bad for you. They clog your arteries and increase your risk for heart disease. Fats that are solid at room temperature are saturated fats, and you should limit them to no more than 10 percent of your overall fat calories. Things like butter, eggs, cheese, and red meat all have saturated fat, so limit your intake of these foods.

Unsaturated fats are good for you. They are heart healthy and will prevent disease. They are liquid at room temperature and are the types of fats you should include most often in your diet. Canola oil, peanut oil, and olive oil all are examples of unsaturated fats and are the ones you should use.

Trans Fats are the enemy! These are liquid oils that have been transformed into a solid fat by injecting hydrogen atoms. Trans fats are found in processed, packaged, and restaurant foods. They have an extended shelf life and are much less expensive for manufacturers and restaurants to use than the other fats. Trans fats increase LDL, decrease HDL, and promote inflammation.

One of those three summaries is true; the others are kinda, sorta true but not really. Trans fats actually are the devil. They are often made from a low-quality oil such as cottonseed or soybean oil, and the chemical alteration creates a molecular structure the body doesn't recognize. These artificially created fats are detected by the body as a foreign substance that must be dealt with, attacked, and destroyed. The inflammatory response kicks in to perform these functions. By consuming foods made with trans fats, introducing foreign invaders, you are in essence, forcing your body into a state of battle, potentially contributing to chronic inflammation.

Let's tackle the idea that saturated fat is bad for you and unsaturated fat is good for you. If you recall, the body breaks down food into the raw materials that make up that food. The fat in food gets broken down into the fatty acids that make up that form of fat. Nearly every food that has fat has saturated fatty acids, monounsaturated fatty acids, and polyunsaturated fatty acids. Whatever it has most of is how the food gets classified (as saturated or unsaturated). Stick with me, I promise I will make this make sense!

There are roughly twenty types of fatty acids found in foods, and the REAL debate to be had is assessing fatty acid vs. fatty acid vs. fatty acid vs. fatty acid. As you can imagine, this is way too complicated, but the problem with lumping them simply into saturated and unsaturated categories is some fatty acids found in foods that have saturated fat are good for you, and some fatty acids found in unsaturated fats are not so great for you. I don't want to get too into the weeds with this, so I will leave you with this simple tip: eat REAL FOOD. Trust nature over chemists. If you can determine with a quick glance the fat came from the Favor These Fats list, I say eat it!

FAVOR THESE FATS
Butter and other Dairy Fats
Coconut Oil and Coconut Butter
High-Oleic Sunflower Oil
Olives and Olive Oil
Avocados and Avocado Oil
All types of Nuts
Oil and Butters from all types of Nuts
Fats from Fish and Footed Animals

FORGET THESE FATS
Vegetable Oil (WHAT vegetable is it made from?)
Canola Oil
Margarine
Soybean Oil (read your labels)
Cottonseed Oil (read your labels)
Any food made with Trans Fats (read your labels)

Dr. Andrew Weil (drweil.com) and Dr. Joseph Mercola (drmercola.com) enlightened me to the facts about fat. They are both great resources should you want to further educate yourself on the truth about fat. I subscribe to their newsletters, which are always full of incredibly interesting and useful information. Join the fun and check them out!

OK, you are going to eat fat, but how much? As a percentage of your overall caloric intake, at least 30 percent, and possibly as much as 70 percent, of those calories coming from fat is a healthy distribution of nutrients. Some of you may be freaking out about the 70 percent, but remember, you are still staying on a calorie budget that is appropriate with your needs and goals (refer to Chapter Two if you need a refresher). If 70 percent of calories are coming from fat, that means you have only 30 percent of your calories to distribute between protein and carbs. Your choices are going to be mostly vegetables and lean sources of protein, since those both come with few calories. Lean protein, real whole-food sources of fat, and lots of veggies—sounds pretty sensible and healthy to me!

A few final thoughts on fat to drive home the point that PFF is your BFF. We have fat-soluble vitamins A, D, E, and K. You need to eat food that has fat when you eat foods that have those vitamins or you won't absorb those vitamins. Let's say you typically go to the vending machine each afternoon for a bag of chips, and in an effort to make healthier choices, you pack carrots to have as your snack instead. Carrots are a healthier choice than chips—no doubt! However, if you eat those carrots by themselves, you will not absorb any of the Vitamin A and, because it is a carbohydrate, the blood sugar will spike then crash—then you'll go get the chips anyway. In addition, you are still going to be hungry and unsatisfied. When we eat fat, it triggers the release of leptin—your satiety hormone. When you avoid fat—most likely in an effort to save calories—you are not getting the benefit of leptin to signal you are satisfied. PFF is your BFF in SO many ways! Have some hummus, cheese, or full-fat ranch dressing (yes, I said it . . . FULL-FAT dressing!) with those carrots. Get on the wagon; I promise it will change your life.

O OR NO?

I am often asked if organic foods are worth the money? Are they really that important? As with most other things, it depends. In the perfect world we would all be eating organic everything. It is probably best to not put toxic chemicals, fertilizers, pesticides, and artificially created substances into the body. These are all deemed harmful, and your body will do its best to get rid of the danger by revving up the immune system and kicking in the inflammatory response. Many healthy people, with optimally functioning immune systems, have the ability to process out all the junk that would otherwise cause real damage. If you have an underdeveloped or an overtaxed immune system, this may not be the case. The amount of junk that is piling in also affects the ability of your body to cleanse itself. The body can only do so much!

In addition, the antibiotics and hormones (naturally occurring and added) found in the food supply can have a seriously detrimental impact on our endocrine system. Recall from the "Know Your Numbers" chapter that your endocrine system is responsible for producing many of our hormones—those chemical messengers that control everything. Ingesting antibiotics through food, as well as the overuse of antibiotics as medicine, can wreak havoc on the body, throwing it severely out of balance.

When considering if you should buy organic, you need to be clear about your own values, beliefs, and health status. Cost is often the reason cited as to why someone is not buying more organic foods. In some cases, the money is well spent, not so much in others. The list of the Dirty Dozen or the Terrible Twenty can help guide you in this decision. These items either have a thin skin, which allows pesticides to penetrate into the food, or they are sweet—which means pests love them. If you are going to invest in organic produce, these will be worth the extra cents. Look for the USDA Organic seal signifying the items have gone through the rigorous testing and have adhered to growing and production standards.

THE DIRTY DOZEN

Apples	Celery
Strawberries	Peaches
Spinach	Imported Nectarines
Imported Grapes	Sweet Bell Peppers
Potatoes	Domestic Blueberries
Lettuce	Kale and Collard Greens

Organic or not, you still need to wash your produce! Running it under water is not washing, so make sure you use either a fruit/vegetable wash or your own solution of one part vinegar to two parts water. This will kill most bacteria and help keep the food from spoiling.

I made the switch to organic animal products years ago when I fully understood the impact antibiotics have on our endocrine system. I believe that minimizing hormonal disruption will reduce my risk for disease and allow my body to function at an optimal level. Where ever you land with your decision on organic, keep in mind that REAL FOOD, even if it's not organic, will provide nutrients the body can use. If the alternative is between processed food and real nonorganic food, I say keep it REAL!

FILLING IN THE GAPS

I am often asked about supplements—are they necessary and do they work? The short answer is *maybe*. Ideally, we are getting most of our nutrients by taking in a wide variety of high-quality, nutrient-dense, whole foods each day. Even if this is the case, we can fall short on some critical nutrients. If you are considering supplements, here are a few important points to think about.

- they will help only if you are deficient or are at suboptimal levels

- you must take them correctly

- they must be bioavailable—in a form the body can use

- they are NOT a substitute for real food (check the definition of supplement)

- they may cause an imbalance with other nutrients

- they may be harmful for you

The aging process, certain health conditions, and taking certain medications may make you a great candidate for supplementation. You really MUST do your own thorough research on any supplement you are considering. It amazes me how many people simply take something because their sister is, or they heard a sound bite about it, or they saw an infomercial that promised magical results. There is no supplement that is going to fix your poor choices! Supplementation in conjunction with the healthy lifestyle, not in lieu of the healthy lifestyle, may be beneficial, but it can be complicated and requires commitment. At this stage in my life, with my current health status and lifestyle choices, I have determined these supplements to be appropriate for ME:

Vitamin D
(almost everyone is deficient or at suboptimal levels)

High-quality omega-3 fatty acid
(for anti-inflammatory effects)

Melatonin
(very low dose before bed)

Rhodiola and Holy Basil
(for adrenal support)

Vitamin B12 spray
(blood tests revealed suboptimal levels)

I imagine at some time in the future I will add glucosamine and chondroitin, and possibly other forms of anti-inflammatory supplements, but for now these are sufficient to fill in the gaps that are nearly impossible to get through nutrition alone and help my body function at a higher level. If you think you could benefit from supplementation, please do your research. Know what each supplement does, be clear about what you are hoping to achieve by taking it, and invest in a high-quality form your body can actually use. If necessary seek professional guidance from a holistic nutritional therapist.

WATER

Because every function in the body requires water, you want to make sure you adequately hydrate each day. If you don't, it must mean there is a drought! To survive the drought, the body will conserve its supply by slowing down every process. It will also have to pull water out of storage from cells and muscle tissue, which means they won't be able to function at capacity. Half your body weight in ounces (a 200-pound person needs 100 ounces of water) is the goal! If you don't like to measure, you can monitor the color of your urine. It should be clear to pale lemonade in color. If it is darker than that, you are dehydrated. We dehydrate overnight through respiration, so a great way to get you going is with 20–30 ounces of ice-cold water. Brush your teeth first (so you don't flush bacteria down your system) and get chugging!

CAFFEINE AND ALCOHOL

Around and around we have gone with these two. Caffeine raises your blood pressure and is bad for you. Wait, no—it's actually good for your brain and helps you focus. Hold up, wait a minute . . . it's linked to early death and gout and causes insomnia. Woot-Woot—it reduces the risk of stroke and type 2 diabetes and some types of cancer. Good golly, no wonder we are all confused! And alcohol—red wine is good for you, right? I mean, if it's good for my heart, it must mean it is a "health" beverage! Sorry, NO! There might be some properties of some types of grapes used to make some types of wine that have some health benefits for some people, but alcohol—including red wine—should not be considered "healthy." Alcohol turns to glucose in the body, causing the spike in blood sugar. In addition, it disrupts the messages the brain and body need to send each other and taxes the liver, which has to metabolize it. I'm not saying you can't include it as part of an overall healthy lifestyle, but to say "it's good for me" as justification for consuming it is just false. It can cause further problems if it is being used as a distraction for dealing with real issues or to create an altered state of mind. Context of use is always important to consider. To enjoy an adult beverage every now and then with friends is very different from needing a few beers (or shots or glasses of wine) to wind down from the day.

With both caffeine and alcohol, your personal health status (such as high blood pressure), specific challenges (difficulty sleeping), and health goals (weight loss) need to be considered when determining how much, if any, is appropriate for you. Frequency, amount, and the context in which caffeine or alcohol is consumed are also important factors to weigh when deciding if these are behaviors you should seek to modify.

YOUR FOOD ATTITUDE

Now that we have covered the basics of nutrition, you may be wondering how you are supposed to get all this healthy food into your body. The first step is to adjust your mindset. The healthy choice is most likely the hard choice, so let's explore a few ways of thinking about food to make the healthy choice a bit easier.

Poison or Medicine

Everything we put in our bodies is either going to promote disease or promote health. The problem is our poison tastes delicious. And it's everywhere, and it's convenient and fun. I think healthy foods taste good, and so far almost everyone I've ever worked with has admitted to liking healthy foods. If it's healthy and you like it, clap your hands. Then eat it!

Reward or Punishment

Have you ever celebrated a birthday with a plate of broccoli? As a child, were you forced to eat your vegetables or there would be no dessert? How we use food creates an attitude about it, and we often see healthy food as punishment and the "treats" as reward. In reality, those treats are punishing your body. It is an act of kindness to reward yourself with high-quality, nutrient-dense foods.

We will cover these concepts further in Chapter Eight as well as explore how your relationship with food developed. For now, I am going to give you some tools to help you start thinking about food in different ways.

Ask yourself, "Am I eating for pleasure or health? What is this food going to do to me and what is it going to *do for me*?" We should enjoy those things we love, but if this is the norm, over time you are slowly poisoning your body. You might not have an immediate negative reaction, but a long-term consequence could show up sometime in the future.

Remember WAITE—Why am I tempted to eat? Simply stopping to ask this question can prevent the impulsive choice you may regret later. This will set you up to start engaging in mindful eating.

A breakthrough for me was when I stopped labeling foods as good or bad—things I was supposed to eat and things I shouldn't. This is dumb. Food is just food. Some foods nourish me physically and help me fit into my jeans, and others feed me a different way—they make me happy in the moment because I love the way they taste. I have to determine what is the appropriate balance of those choices to still end up with an outcome I am OK with. This means I am going to have to have healthy food in front of me so I can put it in my body. If I don't do this, my blood sugar will crash, and by the time I have found food, no matter how great my intentions to make a "good choice," I will choose junk. That's the reality, because once blood sugar crashes, your brain does not have the capacity to think—it has no fuel—so some version of sugar is the only answer to make your brain happy. Although I will love eating that sugar in the moment, I am definitely not going to love the result later!

THE FOUR PS

If you are hiding the healthy food fairy, the one who will drop healthy food in my lap the very moment I need it, please share her! Until then, I have to take care of it myself. I have to Plan, Purchase, Prep, and Pack enough PFF combinations to put in my body every 2–4 hours throughout my day. I do not particularly enjoy this process; there are many other things I need to or would rather do. It's not that fun; in fact, it's hard. Ahh, there it is—it's hard. So why do something I don't really want to? Because if I don't, I'll eat junk. No doubt, I will enjoy those pleasure foods in the moment, but when I can't sleep because my stomach is not thrilled with my choices, I won't be so happy. And when Saturday comes and I can't fit into the outfit I wanted to wear for the party, I'll be mad at myself. And if I do this for years and years, and eventually my doctor tells me I have diabetes, I'll be pissed. That's why. What is YOUR why?

Plan

Start by making a list of healthy foods you like. If you like them, you will eat them! The goal is to make this list as robust as possible so get specific. List all types of nuts and seeds, all sources of protein, all varieties of fruits and vegetables. Don't forget the whole grains, beans, and legumes and definitely don't forget the fat! Get the whole family involved with making the list so everyone is working toward the same goal—healthier eating. Once you have the list, it might be helpful to categorize the foods into carbs, proteins, and fats. I have included a sample list in the back of the book to help guide you. From this list you will start to create PFF combinations that you find appealing and are easy to fit into your lifestyle. Here are a few easy examples:

Apple and hard-boiled egg

Veggies with hummus

Whole grain toast with nut butter and a few banana slices

Roasted veggies (every kind!) in olive or avocado oil with lean meat

Full-fat cottage cheese with a few pineapple chunks

Purchase

The grocery store can be a daunting place, full of confusion and temptations. But there are simple solutions. First of all, bring your list! The list of healthy foods you like serves as your go-to shopping list, and these foods will become staples in your home. If it's not in your house, how are you going to eat it? Too often people shop without really thinking through how and when all their food will be eaten, which ends up with it being tossed out. Proper planning will prevent this, so look at the week ahead to determine how many PFF combinations you need to get you through. There is no need to peruse every aisle just in case there is something you didn't know you needed. Trust me, you'll be OK without it! This is your opportunity to pad your environment for success, so if you know you are going to be tempted to eat cookies when they are in the house, DON'T BRING THEM IN THE HOUSE.

Ideally, most of the things you are buying are real foods with no labels, but if you are buying things that come in a package, it is a great idea to know what you'll be putting into your body. Read and understand the label and ingredients list, even if the front of the package makes it appear it's good for you. The food manufacturers' job is to sell food. They do this by making it taste good for an affordable price, and if they can convince you it is good for you—that's a home run! Although the marketing on the package is legal, it often does not reflect the whole truth.

"I don't have time" is no longer an excuse for not getting food into your house. Almost every grocery store will deliver and at the very least will shop for you and have it ready for pick-up. Take advantage of members-only clubs for huge savings on healthy foods (skip the treats!). If you have a Costco in your area, it is well worth the cost of membership, as you will find nuts, oils, high-quality fresh and frozen fruits and vegetables (many of them organic), eggs, meat, hummus, and dairy products at much lower prices than your conventional grocery store. Even households with few members (one) can benefit, because if you eat the food you buy, you will not be wasting it!

Prep

I think the prep work that has to go into eating healthy is the biggest deterrent for many people. You can avoid a lot of it by purchasing pre-sliced fruits and vegetables. Spend a bit more money but save a lot of time. Or buy the whole foods and learn to enjoy the time you spend preparing them yourself. Either way, the food needs to be ready to eat when you want to eat it. I find it works best to get it home and leave everything out that does not need to be refrigerated. How you found it at the market is how you can store it at home until it has been cut and prepped. Start by washing all produce and let it dry before you package it. If you have a jumble of plastic bags shoved into your crisper drawer, you will not eat what's in them, so use clear containers and keep them at eye level on the shelves in your fridge.

Set aside time on your calendar to do some bulk cooking. My Sunday food prep typically looks something like this:

Make fresh-ground nut butter

Boil 6 eggs

Roast veggies
(usually several of the of the following: asparagus, broccoli,
cauliflower, beets, Brussels sprouts)

Make egg scramble with lots of veggies
(onions, mushrooms, spinach, peppers)

Prepare Crock-Pot or Instant Pot meal (a PFF combo of course)

Pack

Invest in a nice insulated cooler that is large enough to carry all your perishables for the day. Remember, you need to eat most of your calories early and often throughout your day so you will be packing a lot of food. Make sure you have plenty of containers and utensils to get through your week or at least until you can get them washed! I find the eight-ounce water bottles make perfect ice packs. Freeze a few and tuck them in the corners of your cooler and your food will be just fine!

You now know what to eat and how to eat it. Are you ready to embrace this as a lifestyle? You don't have to make all the changes at once—in fact, you should not do that because that will feel like you are on a diet! Here are some things to consider to help with your transition to a healthier way of eating:

1. Expand the list of healthy foods you like.

2. Do a color analysis—write down all your fruit and vegetable intake for one week and circle each with an appropriate-colored crayon or marker. If any colors of the rainbow are missing (remember ROYGBIV?), make a SMART goal

to find foods of that color you can start to incorporate.

3. Embrace PFF as your BFF. Create as many PFF combos as you can from your list of healthy foods.

4. If needed, increase your water intake.

5. Carve out time on your calendar for the Four Ps.

6. Purchase a cooler and storage containers.

7. Practice mindful eating and change the way you think about food.

FINAL THOUGHTS

If you are feeling a bit overwhelmed with all this information, take a deep breath. You are going to be just fine! Pick one thing you are ready to tackle and get started. It has taken me many years to figure it all out, and I am still learning and improving my habits. This is not a race or a competition to see who gets the gold medal for the healthiest eater. All that matters is that you are working to gradually make improvements. One month, one year, or one decade from now normal habits will look very different from how they look today, because you are a Better Being and Better Beings are always seeking to improve. What they don't do is judge, criticize, or sabotage themselves if they are not eating "perfectly." (What does that even mean?) Embrace the process, continue to learn, and be open to trying new things. You may be surprised to discover all the amazingly delicious medicine you've been missing out on!

Chapter Four

MOVEMENT
IS MEDICINE

BY NOW WE ALL KNOW the benefits of exercise, yet somehow it is still not a priority in many people's lives. I am forever grateful for my exposure to gymnastics, because even though we were an active family, sports and exercise were not something either of my parents grew up with. After I quit gymnastics, I had a lot of free time to fill and exercise became the substitute. I felt very comfortable in a gym and around equipment, because I had spent the ages of seven to seventeen in this environment. Before heading off to school in Hawaii, I attended University of Wisconsin–Oshkosh—the same place I spent my life as a club competitive gymnast. I also worked at the front desk at a gym, which was ideal for earning money while I studied for class. The free gym membership and access to it anytime I wanted was a huge bonus. It became my sanctuary, and looking back, I know that exercise was my savior. The gym was one place where I felt 100 percent at ease, not caring what anyone around me was doing or thinking. I didn't look great—mind you, I was already fat—but I knew at the very least I was doing something good for my body. At that point I was not aware of, and could not appreciate, all the good it was doing for my brain and my mental health, but the fact that exercise has been a constant throughout my life, during the good times and the bad, is, without a doubt, the reason I made it out all right. I can only imagine what my years of poor nutritional choices would have done had I never embraced exercise as a lifestyle habit. If I had tossed in the towel and abandoned exercise when stressful life events made things tough, I know my mental health and outlook on life would have suffered tremendously. It is because of my experience, as well as my educational background, that I KNOW exercise is the magic pill for just about everything. The human brain and body were designed for movement. If we stop moving, we stop thriving, then we stop surviving, and eventually we stop living. It really is that simple. My mission is to present to you the power of exercise and to convince you that you cannot, and do not want to, live without it!

Exercise is your best form of preventive care. Think about how much time and money you spend maintaining your home and your car. If you can devote even a little bit of time each day maintaining your body, you will save yourself from a lot of difficult repair later. To illustrate exactly how movement is medicine and magical I am going to detail all the ways it helps us be healthy, high-functioning, disease-free human beings.

HEART HEALTH

Cardio exercise increases the size and flexibility of arteries, which helps to maintain healthy blood pressure. It also stimulates the liver to produce more HDL—the "good cholesterol"—which keeps arteries clean by sweeping up excess LDL. Fat is one of the forms of fuel the body will use to move, and the fat in the bloodstream, called triglycerides, is very accessible. Since these triglycerides are being utilized, they won't be hanging out in the bloodstream causing clogged arteries. Finally, the heart is a muscle and, as with every other muscle, if you don't use it, you lose it. It must be worked to remain strong, and that is accomplished by elevating your heart rate for a minimum of 20 minutes for 3 times a week.

DIABETES PREVENTION

If you are diabetic or prediabetic, or don't ever want to be close to either of those, you MUST exercise. The glucose in your bloodstream is the most readily available form of fuel for the body to use, and if you don't use it, you may eventually build up insulin resistance. Move your body after a meal to immediately use the fuel you just put in!

BONE DENSITY

Up until your mid-twenties, you are building your bone bank—after that it is only withdrawal. Unfortunately, people often do not start to think about their bone density until they discover they have osteopenia or osteoporosis. You cannot reverse bone loss, so it is best to achieve peak bone mass while you are young. Any type of activity that forces you to strike the ground or resist against gravity will help slow down the rate of withdrawal to maintain the bone density, so engaging in regular strength training, walking, running, or jumping activities will do the trick. Activities such as swimming, biking, and using a rowing machine or elliptical trainer, although great for other things, do not help with bone density as there is no contact with the ground.

STRESS MANAGEMENT

Not only does exercise burn energy, but it also helps prevent or reverse a lot of the negative consequences of chronic stress. High blood pressure, cholesterol, and blood sugar can all be results of chronic stress, and we know exercise helps keep these in check. I think the most fascinating way exercise helps manage stress is because it actually serves as practice for all the systems that need to communicate during the stress response. Exercise is a stressor—placing extra demand upon the body—and if you exercise regularly, the hormonal activity and different messages needing to be delivered are the same as when we are faced with an actual stress trigger. You literally are allowing the systems to get in condition so they know exactly what to do when called upon for the fight-or-flight response.

BRAIN HEALTH

Cardio exercise increases the production of brain-derived neurotrophic factor (BDNF). This is produced in the hippocampus and is sometimes referred to as fertilizer for the brain. BDNF stimulates the production of additional dendrites, which are the branches coming off neurons that transmit messages. In addition, these branches grow in length, making it very simple to get the message across to the next branch and down the neurological pathway. A greater number of pathways makes for improved memory and cognitive function. With age, the hippocampus often shrinks, but extra blood flow to the brain will prevent this.

Other types of exercise—anything that challenges your balance or coordination or requires you to "think"—has tremendous positive impact on brain health as well. Your brain has to send messages to your muscles to cause them to move. In the case of balance, when we stand on two feet on solid ground, the muscles in your feet, ankles, and lower legs don't have much to do and the neurons in your brain, which are in charge of those signals, never get to fire. The same is true if we do the same thing all the time and never challenge ourselves to step out of a comfort zone. Anytime you do something new, different neurons are enlisted to send signals to facilitate movement. The more neurons you use, the more you will continue to have—well into your golden years!

INJURY AND CHRONIC PAIN PREVENTION

Poor posture, structural imbalances, or chronic positions can all contribute to pain and injury. Being out of postural alignment will cause some muscles to become weak and overstretched, while others remain constantly contracted. This will result in tightness and a decreased range of motion. Eventually you will compensate your movements, putting other things out of alignment and furthering your risk for injury! Poor ergonomics at your workstation or during other activities can also lead to overuse, eventually resulting in tendonitis or more serious injuries. Sometimes it is simply the way we are designed that leads to issues. Addressing the root cause of the pain and implementing a stretching and strengthening program can help correct these situations, preventing further injury and decreasing the pain.

WEIGHT MANAGEMENT/LOSS

This is perhaps the most common reason people decide to embark on an exercise program in the first place. We know cardio exercise burns calories, so it's a pretty important piece of the puzzle if weight loss is the goal. As important, if not more so, is strength training. I detailed all of this in Chapter Two and will further highlight the magic of muscle in just a bit.

In the perfect world we are all getting a minimum of 10,000 steps a day of movement, strengthening our hearts through cardio exercise 3–6 days a week for 20–45 minutes a day, strengthening all of our muscles 2–3 times a week, and working on our core, balance, and flexibility every day. Do any of you live in the perfect world? If so, I'd love an invitation! If you live in this world, with your reality, and can't possibly do everything you are supposed to be doing, what do you do? Although all aspects of fitness are important, clearly defined goals will help guide your decision about the frequency, intensity, time, and type of exercise in which you engage. Here are some suggestions, depending on your purpose for exercise:

WEIGHT LOSS
Cardiovascular exercise
4–6 times/week
65%–85% MHR
20–45 minutes
Strength Training
2–3 times/week

BONE-LOSS PREVENTION
Weight-Bearing exercise
3+ times/week
Body must be in
contact with the ground
or resisting against gravity

STRESS MANAGEMENT
Any activity that either
burns energy, incorporates
deep breathing or that
you find enjoyable
most days of the week

BRAIN HEALTH
Modest activity
Balance
Coordination

DISEASE
Cardio exercise
3+ times/week
65%–85% MHR
30+ minutes

BONE-LOSS PREVENTION
Cardio exercise
Strength training
Core and Balance
Flexibility

These prescriptions may look a bit daunting, so my advice is do as much as you can, as hard as you can, as often as you can. All-or-nothing thinking is a huge obstacle for many people when it comes to exercise. Have you ever skipped a workout because you were going to get to class late or you didn't have a full hour for the workout? And what did you do instead—probably nothing! Something is always better than nothing. If all you have is five minutes a day, and you work so hard in those five minutes that you are thankful you don't have six minutes, that is better than doing zero. I promise!

Because details matter, I want to clearly outline what each of these terms mean. Too often we are vague in our descriptions and this is how we overestimate what we think we are doing. Understanding these terms is particularly important if weight loss is your goal.

ACTIVITY

Activity refers to any movement you engage in through the normal course of your day. We should be getting a minimum of 10,000 steps per day.

CARDIO: LOW- TO MODERATE-INTENSITY EXERCISE

Low-intensity cardio exercise would be activity that gets your heart rate into the 65–75 percent range of your Target Heart Rate Zone. Anything below 65 percent would be considered normal human activity. Moderate-intensity is 75–85 percent of your THRZ. Remember, you determine YOUR Target Heart Rate Zone based on the formulas in Chapter Two, and the intensity level of a particular workout will be different for each person. Let's say a world-class sprinter is going to go for a walk around the block at a pace of 3 miles per hour. Because of her high level of conditioning, that walk would probably not even be considered exercise, as her heart rate will not be at the 65 percent level. On the other hand, imagine a person who has done nothing but sit on the couch for ten years and maybe is a bit overweight. That same walk around the block at the same pace will definitely be exercise. This person's heart rate will likely elevate well into the 65–75 percent of her THRZ.

CARDIO: HIGH-INTENSITY EXERCISE

When teaching *the You Revolution* class a few years ago, I asked the group, "Who does high-intensity exercise and for how long?" One lady said she did it three times a week for about an hour each time. I challenged her on this, not that I thought she was lying but because I know if it is truly high-intensity, there is almost no way she could do it for sixty minutes. She went on to describe the kick-boxing class she did and how she was breathing hard and sweating like mad, and really killing it. I have no doubt she was working hard, but it wasn't HIGH INTENSITY, and she didn't get to that level the minute she walked in the door, and she didn't stay at that level until the class was over. High-intensity is the 85–95 percent of THRZ. It is awful. It is brutal. It is painful. A person cannot physically work at that capacity for an extended period of time. Which is why we rarely do it. The thing is, it is EXTREMELY effective. Placing such a high demand on your body and all its systems forces adaptation at a metabolic level. The most magical part of it all is after you have finished the bout of exercise, your body continues to burn calories at an accelerated rate for up to 2 hours.

INTERVAL TRAINING

Interval training and high-intensity interval training (HIIT) are great for improving overall heart strength and stamina and for maximizing the use of your time. The less time you have to devote to exercise, the harder you should work during that time. Interval training can be structured in many different ways as you bounce from one end of the THRZ range to the other. I like to do intervals based on my music—sprint during the chorus and back off during the verse. You can go by time; for example, stay at 85 percent for 1 minute and recover at 70 percent for 2 minutes, or stay at 85 percent for 5 minutes and recover at 65 percent for 5 minutes. You can use any modality and either increase the speed or the resistance level to make you have to work harder. If you are walking on a treadmill, keep a steady pace and alter the elevation.

HIIT

High-intensity interval training is currently all the rage. Basically, your interval is between awful and dreadful. Your upper end is around 95–100 percent of Max Heart Rate, then you come to a full rest for a very brief time and go again. Tabata training is a popular form, and it looks like this: All out for 20 seconds, full stop for 10 seconds, all out for 20 seconds, full stop for 10 seconds, etc. You continue this cycle until you can't. If you can do this for longer than 20 minutes, you need to go faster during the "all out" phase.

MEASURING INTENSITY

Measuring heart rate is the most accurate way of determining how hard you are working (assuming you are not on medication that suppresses heart rate!). You can measure heart rate with either a monitor (the ones with a chest strap are most accurate) or by taking your own pulse. When doing a pulse count, count for 10 seconds and multiply by 6 to get your 1-minute heart rate. The first pulse you feel is count 0, not 1. The talk test is a good way to measure—if you can carry on a conversation without getting out of breath, you are either well conditioned or not working that hard. At high intensity there is no way you can even utter a word. Level of perceived exertion is another way to measure intensity. Sitting on the couch eating bonbons (do they even make those anymore?) is a 1 and "my heart is exploding and I must stop this second" is a 10.

STRENGTH TRAINING

Consider strength training if any of the following sound appealing to you:

- independence now and later in life

- reduced risk for injury

- prevention of fat gain or facilitation of fat loss

- increased confidence

- self-defense

I am a huge advocate for strength training for everyone, and I am very thankful I embraced it early on. My evolution with exercise and how I made the switch from cardio central to loving lifting is detailed in Chapter Two, so let me tell you exactly how muscle goes about working its magic. When you strength train, you are actually tearing down muscle fiber. I know it sounds like a horrible thing to damage body tissue, but in this case it's wonderful! When you are in your growing years—up until late teens to early twenties—the pituitary gland is producing the human growth hormone, which is responsible for the growth and cellular reproduction that is occurring. Once we have reached our peak, the production slows down. Although this seems fine since we no longer need to grow, it's not so fine if you want to age well. You see, HGH is also responsible for cellular regeneration, which helps keep us youthful. This is where tearing down muscle fiber comes in—the signals get sent that there is need for repair, which stimulates the pituitary gland to ramp up production of HGH, benefitting us on many other levels than simply repairing and strengthening the muscle fiber.

In addition, repairing this tissue requires a lot of fuel, i.e. calories. Yes, repairing and building muscle fibers burn calories, AND once you have that muscle it will keep requiring fuel to exist! Do you see how magical it is? Another mechanism involves the hormone irisin. This hormone has been studied in recent years, and exact conclusions are not concise, but it appears that this is the "fat-burning" hormone and exercise—specifically high-intensity cardio and heavy strength training—increases the production of it. Irisin is thought to send the message to release the fat you are storing to use as fuel to help repair and grow the muscle you just tore down. If that is not a genius system, I don't know what is. This hormone was only just discovered in 2012 so there will no doubt be much more research to come, but personally I am moving forward with the belief that this is how it works.

OK, you've bought in, right? Now the hard part—you have to do it. And you have to do it correctly. And you have to do it consistently. And you have to do it forever. It's hard—so what's your why?

One reason people don't see "results" is they are not lifting weight that is heavy enough to make a difference. People are so afraid of that word, but in my definition "heavy" simply means you can't do one more with good form. If you pick up a weight and decide to do a few sets of fifteen reps then set the weight down and move on, you might or might not have actually accomplished something. If you struggled to complete the thirteenth, fourteenth, and fifteenth rep of each set, then yes, you worked to muscle fatigue and tore down some muscle fibers. If you could have done twenty, thirty, or forty reps before you couldn't do one more with good form, then unfortunately you didn't challenge your muscles hard enough, which means you didn't tear down the fibers, which means there is no need for repair, which means HGH and irisin will not be produced, which means you will see no change. So, either sit there all day, doing reps with lighter weight until you can't do one more, or pick up something heavier so your sets end by reps eight, nine, or ten.

Ladies are often afraid of heavy weight, thinking it will make them bulky. Muscle is lean and mean—it doesn't take up a lot of space. If you increase muscle mass, but you haven't cleaned up your nutrition, you might not have not shed enough body fat to see the muscle. This could result in a bulky appearance—but it's not the muscle's fault! In addition, women do not have testosterone levels high enough to put on the mass of men. I gotta tell you I chuckle when a lady tells me she just doesn't want to look like a body builder. I PROMISE, your full-body workout a few times a week will not result in you looking like a body builder. Guaranteed! Another thing I hear is, "I don't want muscle; I just want to tone." So, tell me, what is "tone?" It's MUSCLE! It's muscle that does not have a lot of fat covering it up. Yes, you really do want muscle.

There are many ways to build a strength training workout, too many for me to go into in this book. My suggestion, if you are not sure what to do or how to do it properly, is to invest a little of your time and money and hire a personal trainer to get you started. The difference between effective, ineffective, and injury is often a slight change in body position. If you don't know what proper body position feels like, you can't be sure you are doing it correctly. The last thing you want to do is injure yourself, but spending time and energy for no result is not fun either! If you are working out at a gym, take some time to observe the trainers. Are they counters and crickets, trainers who simply count reps or stare off into space, or are they actually training their clients? A good trainer will listen to your needs and your goals and will be able to adapt any workout to adjust for limitations you may have. A good trainer will know how to push you past what you would likely do on your own but also has the sense of when you have reached a limit. A good trainee will communicate with the trainer, will listen to his/her body, and will accept the idea that working out is hard and will most likely be uncomfortable.

You can accomplish a lot on your own as well. My gymnastics coach would often say, "You can always do one more," and this rings in my head nearly every workout! If I truly cannot do another rep with good form, then I have reached sufficient muscle fatigue/failure and can stop. But if I can, I usually do it. There are times I choose not to do one more, even though I could; however, I recognize that if I do that regularly, not only will I stop seeing results, but I will start to regress. Sometimes the "result" is maintenance, which I think is one of the reasons people cut down on the effort they put forth. We can't see maintenance so we think it isn't working. Muscles begin to decondition about 72 hours after you have worked them, so know that consistency is key and really pushing yourself every so often is necessary for changing the outcome!

You don't need a fancy gym, or any gym, to get started with strength training. Remember, something is always better than nothing. If you have a body, you can do body weight exercises. If you have a little bit of space, for less than $100 you can get a variety of resistance bands and other gadgets that can be used for core and balance work to do a workout at home or at the office. . . . Do you love it or hate it when I take away all your excuses? Just wondering.

CORE AND BALANCE

There has been a resurgence lately about the importance of a strong core. Some of the most awful exercises we had to do as part of our conditioning for gymnastics were "the wheel" (now known as the ab roller), wheelbarrow (in a perfect board-like position), and two-person plank lifts (one person in a plank while the other lifts her to a handstand and lowers back down). They were awful because they were hard, but the value of a strong core cannot be understated! For simplicity sake, the core encompasses muscles between the collarbones and the hip bones, front and back. We have become very weak because we have lost the need to use those muscles (how much effort does it take to sit in a chair or on a couch?). If you were never taught proper posture, your muscles have no memory of that position, and the positions we now frequently find ourselves in are resulting in muscle memory that diminishes core engagement.

Working your balance is one way to start increasing core strength. When I would be flailing around on the balance beam trying to prevent myself from falling off, my coach would say, "Be dry spaghetti." Dry spaghetti is tight and tall and in a straight line, quite the opposite of a wet noodle, which is what I guess I resembled at the time. It is nearly impossible to be tall and straight without contracting core muscles—core contraction keeps you in good posture, and good posture keeps your core strong.

The core serves to stabilize your body, which will prevent other muscles from contributing to a movement they have no business being involved in. Core engagement is necessary for reducing risk of injury and for effective use of the muscles you are actually trying to train. Begin engaging your core by being mindful of posture. Start with getting ears, shoulders, hips, knees, and ankles in a straight line. Your chin should be parallel to the floor, ribcage lifted, and shoulder blades squeezed (like pinching a pencil between them). You may need to do a slight pelvic tuck, which is accomplished by contracting your transverse abdominis, the ab muscle that connects one hipbone to the other. This contraction is very simple but may require a little imagination. Pretend for a moment that you have to zip up a tight pair of pants. I know this is going to be tough for most of you to visualize, but play along! You will have to suck up and in to get that zipper up—which will cause the pelvis to tuck under just slightly. It is a very small movement but will bring the spine into a neutral alignment.

Practice this position whenever and wherever you can. Start noticing the posture of others and when you do, double-check yours. I am the posture police of my family—OK, mostly of my parents—and a few years ago while on vacation I noticed a lot of slouching going on. I got tired—well, Mom and Dad got tired—of me harping on them to stand up straight, so instead I just started holding up one finger. (NO, not that finger!) Just my pointer finger as a reminder to straighten up. To most people this looks like I am signaling the number one, and my mom, in a very proud moment, shouted, "I am een." This is the Dutch word for the number one, so now our reminder for posture is the question, "Are you een?"

Chronic neck and back pain is often the result of poor posture, so as core strength increases and posture improves, pain often diminishes.

FLEXIBILITY

As we age, our tendons and ligaments naturally shorten, and the constantly contracted positions we find ourselves in can accelerate the pace. Muscles also become tight and form memory of the positions they are in most often. All of this leads to a decrease in range of motion, which eventually leads to a decrease in mobility. It is critical to stretch the tendons, ligaments, and muscles back to the positions they prefer to be in. Regular stretching is necessary for everyone, because we are rarely going through our days in a straight line. Sitting for extended periods of time (more than an hour) is a common cause of chronic pain and loss of flexibility because it puts many muscle groups into constant contraction. Glutes, hip flexors, quadriceps, and hamstrings become tight, which can start to cause back, hip, and knee problems. If sitting at a computer is your life, you likely experience neck, shoulder, and upper back problems as well. This clearly is not a position the body was designed to be in, so take some time each hour and at the end of your day to stretch.

An exercise routine can also contribute to loss of range of motion if we do not take the time to stretch the muscle out that we have just been contracting. Stretching after the workout or after a particular exercise can keep things mobile and even reduce some muscle soreness.

Yoga, Pilates, or a simple stretching routine that addresses the body parts you need to put back into place can prevent the loss of, and even increase, your range of motion. Again, consistency is important, because you need to ingrain the memory of the position you want your muscles to be in. Stretching will be moderately uncomfortable, but you should be able to hold the position for 30 seconds to 2 minutes. Very gentle bouncing can be beneficial but never stretch cold muscles! Always warm up through a range of motion and ease into a position before pushing some boundaries of comfort!

There it is—the magic pill—all you have to do is take it. If you are ready to embrace exercise as a lifestyle habit—not something you have to do but something you *get* to do—congratulations! If you are already exercising but recognize ways to enhance or complement your workouts, congratulations! Here are some things to consider to make it happen:

1. Define your purpose for exercise.

2. Create a realistic plan that addresses components of exercise most beneficial for your purpose.

3. Carve out time on your calendar and note specifics of what you are doing with that time.

4. Consider an activity tracker and/or heart rate monitor.

5. Kick up your cardio intensity.

6. Lift weights.

7. LIFT WEIGHTS.

8. Pay attention to posture.

9. Make good use of your time—do as much as you can, as hard as you can, as often as you can.

10. What's your why?

FINAL THOUGHTS

If you still are not convinced that exercise is something you can't live without, I have a story that, hopefully, will change your mind. Many years ago, when I was a young personal trainer, a woman came to me asking if I would train her fourteen-year-old daughter. I told her I'd be delighted; we agreed she would bring her in the following week to meet me and talk details. When she came in, what followed behind was a grumpy, slouchy girl with a messy blond ponytail. It was obvious who's idea this was! We decided the plan was to work with me twice a week to improve her overall fitness. I asked Hannah if she had any questions for me, and her answer was, "Nah." Oh, boy, this was going to be fun!

The next time I saw her, she walked in with attitude and a bald head. I commented on what a nicely shaped head she had—clearly not the reaction she was expecting from me. As time went on, Hannah became very comfortable with me and, I dare say, even enjoyed our sessions. I worked her hard each time but also made the effort to get to know her. It wasn't long before she was lighting up the gym with her smile and laughter and her blue hair and quirky outfits. Her nickname became Hannah Pajama if that gives you a clue. Hannah was a kid who felt like everyone was against her and that her parents were the worst people to ever walk the earth. How dare they give her a beautiful home, nice clothes, and every opportunity she could ask for (seriously, how many fourteen-year-olds do you know that have a personal trainer?).

I could tell she was gaining confidence and we started having serious conversations—the ones that are often hard to have and are often never even spoken. She confided in me, and I gave her my word that, unless she was in danger, what we talked about would remain between us. Fast-forward several years, and Hannah is a gorgeous, I mean, stunning, young lady who has morphed into a confident, articulate gal who knows what direction she'd like to head. She became a vegetarian and rode her bike everywhere and is now the friend who is trying to convince her pals to be healthy.

I consider Hannah my biggest success story, and it has nothing to do with weight loss or really any kind of fitness-related goal. I can remember it like it was yesterday. She was on the leg press machine, and we were talking about her trying to get her friend to stop drinking and be healthier. She asked if she could bring her in to work out with us sometime, and I said, "Sure, that would be fun." She then looked up at me and said, "You know you saved my life, right?" This was nearly twenty years ago and it still gets me choked up, but this is the power of exercise. It has the ability to change you in so many ways, so be a Better Being and don't live without it.

Chapter Five

HOW'S THE
CONNECTION?

HERE'S A CHALLENGE FOR YOU: Keep track for one week how many positive, face-to-face interactions you have with another human being. It can be lunch with your best friend or a smile from a stranger passing on the street.

We are pack animals, and hanging with the pack is necessary for physical, mental, and emotional health. Back in the day we were born into a tribe, with each member having a clearly defined role and a sense of purpose and belonging. We were valued and appreciated, and if we were unable to fulfill the role, someone stepped in to help. Obviously, our lives look very different today. As stated many times throughout this book, the environment we are living in is not the one we were created for. I think we are more "connected" yet more disconnected than ever. Are you running with your tribe or away from it? Are you even a member of one? With whom are you sharing positive experiences, creating and strengthening those bonds with each interaction?

Social withdrawal and isolation can lead to a rapid decline in overall well-being. We know babies need human interaction to thrive, and it is well established that the health of an elderly person rapidly declines when they no longer have a socially stimulating environment. For adults, sometimes this isolation is intentional; sometimes it is based on circumstance. We are busy, both physically and mentally, and we are tired! Personality characteristics, life events, and physical location also contribute to how much or how little we are engaging with other human beings.

The relatively recent introduction of, and reliance on, technology has elevated our lack of connection. Seemingly trivial interactions that used to be a regular part of life have been replaced by a more efficient, convenient method. I remember as a kid going to the bank and the post office on Saturday mornings, usually receiving a smile and some kind words (maybe even a sucker or a Tootsie Roll) while my mom or dad had a brief chat with the salesperson. A conversation may even have been started with someone waiting in line. Can you imagine such a thing today? We no longer have need for those interactions because we bank online and use the self-checkout lane at the store. How about this interesting concept—talk to the person in the elevator. Wait, what? Yes! Leave your phone in your pocket and actually speak to the stranger—or person you know—who is standing just a few inches away from you. Each time we pass on the chance to interact, we pass on the chance to release brain chemicals that make us feel good. Dopamine, serotonin, and the bonding hormone oxytocin are all stimulated when we interact with another member of the pack. They strengthen the bonds that say, "Hello, we are both human. We are members of the same tribe and that makes us 'friendlies.'"

MY PEOPLE

The feeling that I never quite belonged started at a pretty young age. I had difficulty finding my tribe or being truly at ease and confident in the role I played in any one group. We all have innate personality traits and are generally classified as introverts and extroverts. I would define myself as an extroverted introvert. I have no problem being social and very much enjoy it, but I also am quite fine being alone. Knowing that I most likely have always been this way helps me make sense of those struggles to fit in, wanting approval from others to be an accepted member of the group. This was one reason I would get upset with my mom when she'd speak Dutch in front of my friends. It made me stand out, and I really didn't like that. Reflecting on this now, it is ironic that I stifled her uniqueness so as not to draw attention to myself. (It is also rather ironic that by writing this book, I am drawing attention to myself!) I think as young people we feel it appears there is something "wrong" with us, if we do not have a huge circle of friends or are not one of the cool kids. In reality we are all just different, not one better than the other, just different.

Unfortunately for many, feeling like they don't belong, and possibly being ridiculed for that, affects self-esteem. Insecurities and mechanisms to cope with those insecurities develop, and it is easy to get drawn into a less than ideal situation. In middle and high school, I was totally under the spell of one of the girls in our group, Crystal. She was a cool kid everyone wanted to be friends with. Crystal lived on a lake and was always inviting people over to have loads of fun, no matter what time of year. I felt so lucky to be one of her "chosen" friends, but little did I know what was really going on. Other people in our group began treating me differently, and she would tell me all the horrible things they were saying about me. Soon Crystal was my only friend, and by graduation I had almost no interaction with many of the others I had grown up with since preschool. It made me sad, especially since she would decide to go days and sometimes weeks without talking to me. I'd be left wondering what I had done wrong, only for her to eventually decide I was again worthy of her friendship. She had a significant impact on one friendship in particular—the one with Jesica, my first friend. Jesica and I grew up a few miles out of town and our parents were good friends. It was her mom who got us all started in gymnastics, and for many years we had a lot of fun together. Jesica also was selected by Crystal to be her BFF, and she fostered jealousy and competition between the two of us. The three of us were friends together, but there was always underlying tension and uncertainty of what position Jesica or I held. It was totally unacceptable for us to be friends without Crystal, and it wasn't long before Jesica and I weren't speaking. A few years after high school, through a mutual friend in the group, Crystal's manipulation was discovered. During the time she had been conveying all the reasons they didn't like me, she was telling them things I supposedly said. Lies. All of it. A very nervous me finally made the call to Jesica. It was a lengthy, emotional phone conversation, and not long after I was reunited with many of the others.

It is astonishing how one person can have that much influence on another, but I was an easy target for Crystal. I think one of the best days of my life was when I realized I no longer needed or wanted her friendship, and I am so happy that, to this day, Jesica is one of my very best friends. Despite the challenges of many years, many states, many homes, and many children, we have both put forth the time and effort to make sure our friendship continues to thrive. I am sure that without having gone through our shared experience, we might not have this strong bond, so I look back on those lost years knowing I learned many valuable lessons. If something doesn't make sense, go to the source and question it. Gossip and assumptions kill relationships and whoever is spreading it has a motive. Having a best friend is great, but it should be someone who builds you up, not one who isolates you from others. Maybe the most significant change resulting from this, was the giant step I took to no longer be a follower. Although these lessons did not occur overnight, they were present and more obvious as I transitioned through friendships during other phases of life. They allowed me to be a better friend and have made me a Better Being.

Although I had difficulty finding a tribe of peers, I was fortunate to have a very positive home environment, one that celebrated and encouraged my individuality. Never once did my parents suggest I play school sports (rather than the private club gymnastics) or pressure me to stay close for college. When it was my turn to have a car (my dad rebuilt VW Bugs for us), I wanted it painted hot pink. It never occurred to me this would make me stand out; it was simply a reflection of my personality that was again a little different.

In many ways my whole family is a bit nonconforming and are all wanderers of sorts. Both of my dad's parents were first generation immigrants, coming over from Germany at young ages. After World War I, at the age of fourteen, my grandfather left the family farm in Bavaria, Germany, and got himself into an apprenticeship for carpentry. He was making cabinets at an abbey near the town of Oberammergau, but that didn't last long. The story is he was caught kissing a nun and got booted, so he had to figure out his next move. He knew real opportunity awaited in America and was sponsored to come to the States at age seventeen, settling in the Bronx. He went to night school to learn English and took as many carpentry jobs as possible. My grandmother came over in her teens with her mother and stepfather but was expected to take care of herself. She was in her late teens when she met my grandpa. By that time he was a superintendent at a boarding house, responsible for all the maintenance work, and my grandma took a job cleaning. In the midst of the Great Depression, they decided it was best to be self-reliant rather than surviving on the scraps they were getting in the city, so with the money they saved, they bought a small farm in a tiny town called Kripplebush in New York. Earning a living as an egg farmer was hard. Really hard. They worked 24-7 to provide for their three kids, and they set high expectations for their children. There was little time for fun— school and work on the chicken farm took up every minute. My grandparents did the best they could, but I imagine it wasn't the greatest childhood experience for any of them.

My dad left home at seventeen to join the Air Force and set himself up for a different life experience. He took night classes and extra jobs at every opportunity and jumped at the chance to be stationed overseas. When he landed in The Netherlands, he met my mom. At the time she was a sassy Dutch girl, living the good life with her high-class European upbringing, but this American soldier changed all that. It was always her destiny to come to America and at twenty, she left the comforts of home to come to a foreign land. They worked hard to put my dad through school and moved to Massachusetts for his first job. Along came Nicolle then a move to Racine, Wisconsin, where I was born. A few years later they moved ninety miles north to the little town of Winneconne, where we lived throughout childhood.

My mom is a strong personality and an independent thinker who is not afraid to voice her ideas. At the same time, people flock to her because she is thoughtful, helpful, and caring. She is quite the go-getter and the one who awakened my entrepreneurial spirit. My parents made the decision to have my mom stay home when we were young, so she was a rare nontraditional student, going through night school while I was in gym practice. She had a plant business (think Tupperware parties for plants), and I had so much fun being her helper. She eventually made her way into the corporate world, putting her sales skills and languages (fluent in five!) to use. At the time, international sales was a pretty novel concept in her industry, but she was determined to prove herself worthy. She faced a lot of challenges, not only being a woman in a power position but also being foreign in a homogeneous environment. Her robust personality and opinions were not always well received. Ultimately, she chose her values over a paycheck and eventually went into business for herself selling real estate.

I give this backstory because it makes it so clear why my parents raised us the way they did. My dad often says he took the best parts of his childhood experience and tried to copy them for us. The things that made him want to run away from home were what he did the opposite of. There were high standards set and a bit of discipline (all totally justified!), but also there was a lot of love, support, and fun and incredible experiences most kids never have.

One of the many things I am tremendously thankful for is that my parents never compared me to my sister or vice versa. There was one particular teacher in high school who did this ("your sister never struggled with math; I don't know why you can't get it"), but I think because I was so used to being different, it actually had little effect on me. If anything, it probably made me want to differentiate myself even more, and it is true . . . my sister and I are very, very different. Neither is better than the other; we are equally great—just different!

Nicolle is much more of an extrovert and was involved in everything in high school—cheerleading, band, choir, forensics, and probably a few more I am missing! She has always been very social, where for me it requires dedicated effort to make sure I stay engaged rather than just staying comfortable hanging out at home. She tends to be much more of a worrier and a perfectionist and sometimes has a hard time of letting go and moving on from things. Being the big sister, Nicolle was always worrying about me, and at times in our lives she felt I handled certain situations better than she did. This actually caused a great deal of tension between us. I didn't understand why she felt she didn't measure up, and I'd get frustrated and annoyed with her. From my side, she was amazing: captain of the cheerleaders, valedictorian, dancer extraordinaire, the better cousin/niece/granddaughter, and she was forging new paths as a female in a highly male-dominated career field (astrophysics—seriously!)

We were not very close during our teens and into young adulthood. There are many reasons why sisters don't get along, but I think part of it was we did not fully appreciate that we could be different yet equal. Over time, and through patience and deciding that our relationship as sisters and friends was important, we have become closer than ever. There were several circumstances that could have resulted in a serious rift, and I am so grateful we both had the desire to gain a better understanding of the other to prevent that from happening. It required hard conversations, patience, and constant work on both our parts, but we now enjoy a strong friendship and genuinely like each other. At times, I didn't think this could even be possible, and I know a lot of siblings don't make it to this point. I give credit to my parents for never playing favorites and allowing us to thrive as individuals. They also instilled the belief that we had to get along because we are all we truly have. You don't get to pick your family, and I know I am lucky I was born into the one I was, but the nurturing environment played as big a role as anything else. I think having been exposed to so many experiences and cultures at a young age allowed me to gain a broad perspective and appreciation for differences I would later encounter.

RELATIONSHIPS

Throughout life we will be part of many different relationships. Some we are born into, others happen due to circumstance, and many are intentionally fostered. There are some we really want and some we feel we are supposed to have. Regardless of the genesis and the specific nature of these relationships, there will always be a beginning and an end (at least in this life), with some degree of ups and downs in the middle. I am going to skip right to the end of relationships, because it is often this phase that presents a fair amount of difficulty for many people.

Breaking up is hard to do and probably something nobody actually enjoys. Whether it is a significant other, sibling, parent, friend, or an employer, at some point you may realize the healthy option is to move on. It's hard, which is why many people stay in situations they know are not working. The misery you know is easier than the difficult process of ending a relationship followed by the transition to a new situation. In addition, you may have to be part of the other person's process. If you have reached the point where you are ready to make this choice, be kind. Keep in mind you have most likely gone through many of the stages of processing, but for the other person, this is all brand new. Be patient and compassionate but be clear. Sending mixed messages in an effort to not "hurt" the other party is going to result only in confusion, frustration, and anger.

Sometimes the decision is made for you and, whether you agree with it or not, it's happening. This was the situation I found myself in nearly three years into my marriage. To set the stage for stories I will share in Chapter Six, I will sketch a very condensed version of my life with Travis.

"You should probably walk away right now. I'm really, really damaged." Travis said those words to me four hours into our first date. I knew two hours prior that I would never willingly leave this man. At thirty-five, I was a happy, independent, confident, moderately successful girl content with my life. After several long-term relationships with men who clearly weren't "the one," I had grown to understand what I wanted in a partner. I did NOT want to spend my life alone, but I knew I'd rather be alone than with the wrong person. My parents set a very high standard for marriage, and if I didn't have that, I didn't want it at all. In the summer of 2007, through rather random circumstances, Travis entered my life. What happened on that first date is honestly inexplicable. The best way I can describe it is there was a major shift of energy, and it propelled us both into existing in the same time and space with each other. (Get your minds out of the gutter—it's nothing like THAT!) We spent eight hours talking, and it truly was like we had known each other forever. Believe what you will about past lives, spirits, energy—this connection was like nothing I had ever experienced.

The next day I went to the gym as usual, but it was as if I had landed on a different planet. I literally had no idea what I was supposed to do there and wandered around aimlessly, my brain completely absent. I couldn't think of any exercises to do and even the machines were foreign objects. I saw several clients that day—all of them waiting anxiously to hear about the date. I couldn't tell them anything. Not because I didn't want to but because no words would come! Later that evening I hung out with Lisa. She wanted details, but formulating a coherent sentence was impossible. It was the most bizarre sensation ever—one that has never been duplicated. And it was mutual. From that day on Travis and I spent almost every free minute together. He used to tell his version of how we met and how he recognized about three weeks in that he realized he was in love with me by day three. We had a lot of fun but also spent a great deal of time talking about the challenges he has faced since a young age. None of what he told me came as a surprise. In fact, on that first date, when he told me to walk away, I instinctively had a clear picture of the daily struggles going on in his head. It didn't scare me, and it wasn't a red flag, but it was just part of his makeup. The internal demons were no match for all the incredible qualities I saw in him, and there was nothing to fear. I knew with the right environment and a person who was well equipped to help him manage these struggles it would be just fine.

It was more than just fine—it was amazing. I belonged! I found my person, and it was incredible. We were engaged within a few months and married nine months to the day of our first date. We were "that" couple who were so completely meant to be together, and apparently it showed. At a charity event with my good friend Jen and her husband, Chris (Travis's favorites of all my friends), a total stranger came up to us to say she had been watching from across the room and loved the energy she was witnessing between the two of us. She said we had something rare and special, and she hoped we made sure to never let it end. Some in our circles were ecstatic, others were skeptical, and a few were completely unsupportive. Some of my closest friendships became strained, and it became increasingly unpleasant to be around those people. Gradually, we drifted and those bonds weakened. I was heartbroken at the deterioration of what I thought were strong friendships, but my husband and my marriage would always come first.

Not long into our marriage, the economy plummeted. Travis was a financial advisor and I was self-employed, and we owned a few rental properties. Everything in our world took a hit and, financially, times were quite tough. This situation proved to be a significant trigger for him, and deep dark days followed. I knew we would be fine—I had plenty of savings and we are both intelligent, resourceful people—but his confidence and self-worth took a major blow. On the outside he was the funny, charming, kind human many people knew, but on the inside, he loathed everything about himself. There was rarely an issue with "us," but he spent so much time hating himself and even more time hating himself for not being a better husband and provider, that I eventually became a manager of his emotions. What we did or did not do was predicated on how he was feeling that day. I truly was fine with whatever we did, because when we were together, I still felt fulfilled. Even through his most difficult battles, he cherished me. He was the guy who had the eight-by-ten wedding picture on his desk at work and who bragged to all his coworkers about how lucky he was to have such an amazing wife. He would regularly tell me, "You, my dad, and my brother—you are the constants in my life. No matter what, the three of you will always be in my life and I will do everything I can to protect you." At the time, I had no idea how true those words would be but not exactly in the way I thought.

So now I fast-forward to spring of 2011. I knew Travis's tells. Growing a full beard, listening to Christian music, spending more time on Facebook, and reaching out to certain people were some of the signs I recognized as patterns when he was in a bad place. A few other things were swirling around our lives at this time, and I sensed he was really fighting hard against his internal demons. May 11, 2011, is when those demons finally won. I arrived home from training a client late in the afternoon to find him sitting on some chairs in the lobby area of our hallway at the condo. I knew instantly something really awful had happened, but I was completely unprepared for what came next. That is actually a severe understatement, but I don't even know how to put it into words. He told me that he couldn't do it anymore. He was tired of his constant struggle and just didn't want to continue fighting. He proceeded to tell me I was the best thing that had ever entered his life, I was the most incredible wife ever, and I was the reason he had lasted this long; for him to survive going forward, however, he needed to leave me.

As you might imagine, this made absolutely no sense to me. It was clear that this was not my husband talking, and no decisions were going to be made until we got him some help. Unfortunately, the only way to get immediate help is to check into a hospital psych ward. This was a devastating experience for us both, but it also offered a glimmer of hope. For the first time, he felt like he would find some answers and maybe eventually feel "normal." Over the course of the next few months, my priority was to make sure he was going to be OK. I moved through this time with only his well-being in mind. After the hospital he came to feel his survival required him to be on his own. Apparently, I did too good of a job "taking care of" him, and he just needed to feel like he was capable of taking care of himself. I supported him in his decision to move out, but I asked of him, "Whatever you do, please surround yourself with healthy people who have nothing but your best interests at heart." He promised that he would.

It was a shaky few months to say the least, and by the end of summer, he decided divorce was the answer. With his ongoing process of figuring out treatment and medications, I felt like this was still not a time for major decisions. We basically stopped communicating and since I was not going to initiate the end of our marriage, I carried on as usual. One day in late October I received an email from Travis. This was the first of several "apology" emails he sent over the next few years. I had always told myself that if at some point he reached out, realizing he made a huge mistake, I would be willing to see if we could salvage our marriage. I knew this email was him knocking on the door to see if I'd open it, so after several months of silence and a brief email correspondence, we finally spoke on the phone. He had a lot to tell me about the few months we had been apart—none of it pleasant. In short, all the things he said he was going to do—dedicate himself to the healthy lifestyle, surround himself with positive people, stay away from alcohol and anyone with ulterior motives—he did the complete opposite. He laid everything out on the table, knowing that if we were going to be back together, he had to be completely honest about all his goings on. He was embarrassed, ashamed, and remorseful, and honestly didn't even know why I ever would forgive him and want him back. It was something I was going to have to seriously contemplate, but I also believed that those were the actions of someone other than the man I married. I decided to proceed with the belief that you can't compete with crazy and to chalk up the past few months to his truly not being of right mind.

Before moving forward, there were a few loose ends he needed to tidy up, and while all that was happening, I reflected on our life together. I knew we had a huge mountain to climb, but I have read stories of people who have gone through similar situations. With commitment and hard work and both wanting the same outcome, it is possible to come back better than before.

This was my attitude going into it, and my eyes were wide open. We sought out a therapist and worked to reestablish trust. He also had a tremendous amount of work to do on his end, as living with a pretty significant mental health issue is not easy. There is no quick fix and it requires constant dedication to continue to make healthy choices in all aspects of life. This means regular exercise, healthy food, staying away from alcohol, and getting plenty of sleep. It also means self-regulating when you recognize negativity and anxiety creeping in. These are difficult things for almost anyone, but they are absolutely critical for a successful outcome if you are also dealing with mental health challenges. I, too, had some work to do to better understand how to support without enabling. Looking back, I now know that my "taking care of him," something many husbands only dream of, was in his eyes making him feel inadequate. My managing emotions and situations to make it easier for him only served to reinforce his behavior. I would need to learn to walk these lines very carefully.

About four weeks into therapy, and speaking to and seeing each other regularly, there was a noticeable shift. He was not texting and emailing as much, and when we spoke, he was brief and distant. It doesn't take a genius to know what was happening. If Travis was not talking to me, he was talking to someone else. One serious trigger for him was, he couldn't deal with someone being "mad" at him. The thought of a person hating him was his worst form of punishment. I had a pretty good idea who he was talking to, and after my suspicion was verified, I knew what I had to do. Our next therapy session was just a few days away, and I would be ending things for good. It was quite theatrical (I can totally see it played out on the big screen), and eight minutes into our session, I thanked the therapist for her time, wrote her a check for the session, and walked out. A few weeks prior, the response to him from one of the loose ends he needed to tidy up was, "Go fuck yourself." After I left the room, I opened the door back up for a few final words . . . "and Travis, I agree with Kendall—you can go fuck yourself."

Those were the last words I ever intended to speak to Travis. It was obvious to me therapy was just a charade. It was his way of appearing to try to save our marriage, when in reality it was simply for him to make sure I didn't hate him. Well, he failed. I hated him with every ounce of my energy. The line between asshole and mental illness is very blurry, but this was definitely on the side of asshole. Gone was any shred of empathy or compassion I had for this person. To move forward, I carried on as if the last four years never happened. I wanted to know nothing about him and asked everyone in my circle to never speak his name or of our time together. He no longer existed to me and I was going to be just fine. Those friends who were skeptical and unsupportive of our relationship in the first place were there to swoop in and take care of me. My family was nothing but wonderful, even though they knew very little of what had been going on. I sheltered most of my family from much of what happened, not only to protect them but to protect Travis too. Despite what he had become and all the pain he had delivered, I never wanted to cause him pain in return. Funny, even then, I was still compelled to take care of him.

All that transpired was so completely out of character with what I knew about the man I married. The same person could not have lived both lives. So either everything about my relationship with him prior to May 11 was a sham or this period of time was. I knew for a fact what I had just gone through was real, so that left little choice—our life together was a big fat lie. I believe from our first date on, Travis said and did whatever he needed to say and do in the moment to meet his needs. There is no way he actually loved me the way he said he did. There is no way that I meant to him what he said I did. "You, my dad, and my brother—the three constants in my life." What happened to that? Me, the ONLY person in his life who never judged him, never diminished him, did nothing but love and support him in every way, and who sacrificed a lot of her own needs and wants—this is what you do to that person? Travis was really only concerned about Travis. Everything he said or did was so he felt OK with himself. This was an ugly truth for me to uncover but one I firmly believed. I wish I had never met him. The way it ended dwarfed all the amazing times we had, and I certainly didn't need to go through it. Now that it was officially over, I could get on with my life. Life was great before him, and it would be just as great without him. He did me a huge favor and probably actually did "protect" me like he always promised he would, for it would not have been an easy life. In my mind we were done and done. As you will see in the next chapter, I was wrong—REALLY WRONG!

From a physical and emotional standpoint, I did come out of this time fairly all right. True friends come out during your toughest times, and it was humbling for me to see what amazing support I had all around me. It wasn't easy nor was it always smooth, but I did my best to take care of my critical needs. Managing stress through change is one of the hardest things to do, and my advice is always going to go back to the basic elements of self-care. Put high-quality food in your body, move your body, get the best sleep you can, surround yourself with healthy and positive people, and incorporate some element of mindfulness to redirect your mind away from negative thoughts. Remember, YOU CONTROL YOU and that's all. If change is happening, choose to proceed through it in the healthiest, most positive way possible. You might not understand it, but I have learned we are not meant to understand everything, and although it is not your choice, trying to make sense of it will be a waste of time and energy. I have met few people whose lives have turned out exactly as they planned, and the sooner you can move past hard times, the more time you'll have to enjoy the next great thing.

GET OUT!

After navigating through the difficult time with my divorce, I decided that my motto for the year was to "not be so lame." I used to lead a rather fun, interesting life, but found that I had stopped doing things because I just didn't want to be out there. I was actually fine being boring, but I know that's not healthy. In an effort to not be so lame, I became proactive in being the friend who reaches out to make plans rather than waiting to see if anyone invited me along. Concerts, shows, sporting events, weekend trips—all things that take planning. A simple dinner and a night of trash TV with my best friend was, and still is, one of my go-tos, just to get out of the house and not be alone. My most recent motto for this year is to "explore and expand." To say yes, when I would instinctively say no and to step a bit further outside my comfort zone.

I still am perfectly fine being alone, and in many ways, it is much easier, but there is a lot of fun to be had when you interact with other human beings. At this point in my life, I am quite picky about who I spend my time with. A person must add value in some way or I will probably pass. I don't look for other people to fill a void but rather to complement the great life I have. I find that people who tell me I HAVE to meet someone are usually reflecting their own desire to not be alone. They truly can't comprehend how anyone would be OK (more than OK!) going through life without someone constantly at their side. I realize it is healthy to have quality relationships, but I also believe it is healthy for those who "can't be alone" to work toward a place where they are comfortable and capable of self-reliance. One way is not better than the other—they are just different—and healthy balance is what each of us should define for ourselves and strive for.

Another avenue of exploring and expanding was to get more involved with my community, a beautiful high-rise complex near downtown Denver with a whole bunch of amazing neighbors! I started talking to the people I would see in the gym every day and was usually the one to ask someone's name after seeing them on several occasions. I now also try to attend the social activities and to have conversations with people at the pool. We live by a beautiful park with ample opportunity to head out for a walk with a neighbor; all it takes is a little planning. These relationships with people in my immediate environment are so beneficial to me. It is easy to fall into the pattern of getting in the house and never emerging until absolutely necessary, and with my odd schedule I could go days without crossing paths with anyone. Some of you may think this all sounds silly, but believe me, it is much easier to stay anonymous and NOT to engage! The hard choice has made me a Better Being.

COMMUNICATION

Poor communication, whether it is a difference in style, a difference in interpretation, or simply a lack of it altogether, is often at the root of some of our challenges. Have you ever found yourself in an argument because what you understood was not what the other person meant? Sometimes the expectation has not been clearly articulated and can be interpreted in several ways. Or my favorite—that someone else should just KNOW what I am thinking! One thing is clear, ineffective communication leads to more time, energy, and money being spent than is necessary, and the end result is increased stress! As I navigated through my personal and professional life, I have been exposed to a variety of communication styles, and once I recognize tendencies of a certain person, I find it helpful to adjust my delivery. My favorite example of this happened with my friend Brandon. Let's just say Brandon has a different idea of how the world should run—without time constraints. A few years back we were out for a bike ride, and I asked him what time it was. After a quick glance at his watch he told me it was eight o'clock. It felt to me as though we had been riding for much longer than twenty minutes, so after about a minute I asked him, "Exactly what numbers are currently appearing on your watch? And please read them from left to right." His reply, "eight, one, seven." In his world, if it has an eight in front of it, it is eight o'clock, but in my world the minutes actually matter. I used to get frustrated with Brandon, because whether you believe the world should run on time or not, IT DOES! I can't change him, but I can change my approach to how I communicate with him and resolve the issue.

I have had clients who often take things literally (they are usually doctors and engineers), and this has led to some interesting situations in the gym. On one occasion I was having my client do bicep curls on one side while sitting on a fit ball. After she completed the reps on her right arm, I told her to "shift your weight." She looked at me quizzically then adjusted her sitting position so that ALL her weight was over to one side (while continuing to hold the dumbbell in her right hand). We still joke about it many years later. These are funny, harmless examples, but they highlight for me how easily things can go wrong when a misunderstanding occurs. They have made me more mindful of my words, requests, and instructions. I also make sure to check myself first if someone may not have understood what message I was attempting to convey rather than deciding they are dumb, rude, or intentionally disregarding me.

In many ways technology has made it easier to deliver messages but more difficult to interpret them! The pressure to respond immediately simply because the capability exists contributes to the challenge. Do you get annoyed when someone hasn't immediately responded to your text or email? Do you ever fire off a quick response only to realize you didn't answer the question that was asked? Or maybe sent it to the wrong person or said some things you would like to reel back? Yes. Yes. And Yes. Unless your job requires you to be on call 24-7 and to respond to a crisis in a moment's notice, you will survive without being constantly connected. Think about it: somehow our parents made it without technology!

I feel social media in particular has led to a serious decline in our need and ability to communicate. When Facebook first came out, I was as enthusiastic as anyone else, but I soon found that I was no longer calling my long-distance friends to see how they were. Getting together with local friends was becoming rare as well. Why would I go through all that effort when I can just look at the Facebook feed and know every single thing that is going on in their lives? In an effort to keep up with everyone, I quickly realized I knew no one. It didn't take long before I decided social media was not for me. I would rather have five real friends than 500 FB friends, because it really is about quality not quantity. A quality relationship takes time and effort, and spending energy on too many FB friends means my real friendships might not thrive. Who will be there in a crisis or be the ones you first think to call when you have exciting news? Focus most of your energy here to nurture relationships that matter and let go of those who are no longer serving a healthy purpose. As long as it is reciprocal, where both parties see value, the friendship will be worth the time and effort.

I only recently resumed my social media use (with a great deal of resistance!) because of my business. Being an introvert, and never really liking the spotlight, it makes sense that I am not a huge fan. I once again find myself not quite fitting in. When I look at posts from others in my industry—how beautiful their food pictures look, how they know exactly the right words and emojis to use, and how they have hundreds of "likes" and followers—I recognize how amateurish mine are. The difference between before and now is I DON'T CARE! It is such a beautiful feeling to simply be comfortable with who and what you are. I do my best to post helpful, thoughtful information, but I try to spend as little time and energy as possible worrying about what it looks like compared to others.

There is now plenty of evidence that suggests social media is detrimental, not only to the quality and strength of relationships but also to one's self-esteem. Feeling the pressure of "the perfect post" is not unique to me, and the constant comparisons we make regarding what other people's lives appear to be, often leave us feeling inferior. Don't get me wrong; there are definite benefits to social media. I love seeing the interesting and inspiring things people I know are doing. It is wonderful for keeping up with the changes happening with family and friends—especially the children. But I know many people who have a hard time being happy when they see others succeed. Someone else's success—whether real or staged for social media—has no real impact on your life, but it can stir up judgment or jealousy, which are great instigators of the pity party! Some find it challenging to use social media ONLY for the positive aspects. It is quite easy to get sucked down the rabbit hole of negativity—a huge waste of time and energy—especially when you consider it is effectively changing nothing! If you find this to be the case, I encourage you to establish some boundaries for yourself, maybe limiting who you follow or how much time you spend each day. If you recognize that you are obsessed with how many likes and comments your posts are getting, consider reducing how often you post. Check yourself if someone else's news causes you to feel inadequate and determine what steps you can take to move past that. Of course, you should continue to use it for good—follow me on Facebook and Instagram—just don't judge me by the quality of my food photography!

JUDGMENT

Brief communication is another reason I find social media—especially for my business—to be so challenging. There is no way you can convey complete and accurate information in a short sentence. The soundbite or headline is all that gets noticed and, in my opinion, this is why there is so much confusion! The short answer is almost never the full answer, but people can't seem to find time or patience to actually listen to the whole explanation.

In so many cases context, background story, or just detailed information is necessary to fully understand and make an informed decision. I just saw an ad on TV that epitomizes this. It is a woman walking with her bag over her shoulder and talking on her cell phone. She passes a young man standing up against the side of a building with his hood up. Then you see him bolt after her and grab onto her bag. Horrible, right? He's about to rob her, and you assume the commercial is a PSA about safety and knowing your whereabouts. But then you see that she was about to step into the street to cross and a truck was barreling down her path. The young man jumped in to pull her to safety. The ad is actually a PSA about judgment! Do you ever judge a situation or make a decision without knowing the whole picture?

I committed long ago to giving a thoughtful, thorough answer, not the easy answer, and that also extends to my decision- and opinion-making process. I encourage you to not settle for the simple explanation and to not form opinions based on one side of a story. Once well-rounded information has been gathered, it is up to each of us to decide what aligns with our beliefs and values. Sometimes we think a person is not understanding what we are saying, when in reality, they understand, but they just don't agree. And THAT IS OK! Many things shape our beliefs, and often there is not one that is right and one that is wrong. We can even be kind to people we disagree with. By a certain age or due to particular life events, most people will not be swayed to the other side through arguing. However, the ability to recognize another's point of view as valid is healthy and necessary for a positive environment. If one party is not willing to acknowledge that an alternative perspective may have merit, it is best to steer clear of the topic or the person.

WHAT'S YOUR PURPOSE?

Without a sense of purpose, there is little reason to get up in the morning. At certain times in life your purpose is inherently established, and at other times it might be unclear. Perhaps your purpose is to be a parent, a good friend, or a provider. You may identify it by your career path or a cause you are passionate about. However it is defined, it is clear that a human being needs purpose in order to thrive. Depending on your current situation, this may or may not be something you need to address, but know that as you transition through life, you will find yourself facing this question. At some point your relationship status might change, you will become an empty-nester, and you will probably eventually retire. Perhaps an evolution of values and beliefs may steer your purpose in a new direction. Stagnation is a horrible thing and will soon leave you feeling like that murky, stinky standing puddle. You are never really floating—always either swimming or sinking. The pace can sometimes be undetectable, so you think all is well, but when you notice you are unmotivated, antsy, or generally apathetic, it is a good idea to check in and get moving. To stay engaged in your life you need to be challenged, and that feeling of accomplishment is very motivating.

I've been present through many of these experiences with myself, friends, and clients, but the most astounding example was with my father. He was nearing retirement, and the plan for many years had been to retire in Hawaii. We had been vacationing there since the early 1980s, and my dad was fortunate enough to frequently visit for work. Of course, it was near and dear to my heart, having gone to school at UH, so I was thrilled when they bought a home and were ready to make the move. They had several contacts on the island and soon became involved with their new community—a lovely mixed-dwelling environment near the ocean and on a golf course. It was, however, quite a change. They had begun to downsize a few years prior, out of the country home I grew up in and into a smaller place in town, but this was high-density living in a high-density city! Mom and Dad got right after it, remodeling every room in the house, but as the projects were winding down, the apathy set in.

My dad is a pretty happy guy by nature, but you would have thought they had been deposited into a Third World country with no hope in sight for a happy life. Nothing was further from the truth, but in my dad's mind, there was not a single redeeming quality about where they were. There were definitely challenges: the family dog was in her final months of life, my mom's bad knees made walking difficult, and even in Hawaii traffic is traffic! During one of my visits it was obvious to me my dad was struggling with all the changes and with having lost a main part of his identity. Not only was he no longer working, but he also was no longer traveling and interacting with a lot of different people every week. He was not greeted by the familiar faces at the various airports and hotels he frequented. He had really enjoyed what he did, was very good at it, and was appreciated for it—all of which ceased when he retired. My dad is a doer. He is not a hobby guy but has to always be producing something. This is a great trait to have as long as there is something to produce. With the wrap-up of the home projects, he had no purpose, and it was clearly affecting his attitude, emotions, and energy.

I won't go so far as to say I saved my dad from going over a cliff, but . . . kind of. On a long walk around the gorgeous property, I helped him brainstorm about what was next. Is there a part-time job that interested him? Maybe there were volunteer opportunities he'd enjoy. What about a consulting gig in his previous profession? Every suggestion was met with some variation of no. But I obviously stirred up some thoughts, because after we were back at the house, I saw him busy on his computer. He was doing research to see what was out there for service trainings in hydraulics (his area of expertise). It turns out there is a rather large company based in Denver, and he sent an email and his résumé. He received a response right away, saying he sounded like a perfect fit to teach classes throughout the year on a contract basis. Knowing it is not financially sound to spring for flights from Hawaii, it was suggested that he check in should he ever find himself back on the mainland. Soon after that correspondence, my dad had another conversation with a former industry contact and was offered a job if he ever found himself back in Wisconsin.

To say he "found" himself there is not quite true. The decision was made to move back, and in less than six weeks they had the house packed and a tenant ready to move in. My mom found a short-term rental for them while negotiating on a home she had her eye on. Start to finish, retirement in Hawaii lasted less than eighteen months, and back to Wisconsin they headed. The change in my dad was nearly instant, and they have made a new home in a small town about an hour from where I grew up. My mom is again the social butterfly of the neighborhood, organizing get-togethers and being the first to welcome a new neighbor. They have completely remodeled the house, including a third garage and an overhaul of landscaping. And when I say "they," I mean my mom and dad did it themselves! They also built a "we shed" on some property we've had forever WAY out of town. In addition, Dad is working part time in the summers at one of his former dealers and does six to eight service schools per year all around the country. Mom keeps herself busy with sewing projects, the garden, the house, and her social activities. There is plenty of time for travel—whether it is to warm up in Aruba or Hawaii, chill in Germany, or explore something completely new down in New Zealand. The visits to me and my sister typically revolve around some type of project, and I am truly blessed to have these wonderful people for parents! The decision to leave Hawaii was not easy. Moving there came with great effort and expense, and some would see leaving as a failure—the failure to retire correctly. Although I personally wish they still lived there, I am happy they have found the place they can thrive, and I know that the move back to Wisconsin was a good thing for all of us.

So, fellow human, how are you right now? Have these thoughts inspired you to do something to strengthen bonds or button up your communication skills? Have you been treading water and are ready to start swimming? If you feel that enhancement in your connections, communication, or purpose will make you a Better Being, here are some things to consider:

1. Reflect on the relationships that are truly important to you and assess if you are spending your time and energy accordingly.

2. Set boundaries around your social media use.

3. Be more thoughtful about your communication—both sending and receiving.

4. Be a well-rounded gatherer of information before you make a decision or form an opinion.

5. If you are in a state of transition, clearly define your purpose.

6. Make a new friend.

FINAL THOUGHTS

You've had plenty of my thoughts in this chapter, so I want to close out with just a few more words about friendships. "Make new friends, but keep the old. . . ." This song lyric is one of my favorite lessons from my time in Brownies. People will pass in and out of your life, and all along the way you may need to decide if a friendship is worthy of your time and energy. Likewise, people will be deciding that about you. Given all the demands and various stages of life we go through, forging new friendships in adulthood can be challenging. A few friends I have had for years like to tease me when I start talking about a new one. For some it is not necessary—perhaps you already have a diverse circle or your large family lives close by—but for me, making new friends is extremely important. I live far from where I grew up and have no family close. I don't have the type of job that provides a built-in social network, so knowing only a handful of people, who are all very busy with their lives, would mean I am alone most of the time. A new friend does not diminish the importance of old ones, but it does require effort to find the time and energy to nurture them all.

I understand that, much like flowers, friendships require different types of care. There are many people who have been in my life for a long time, and regardless of whether it has been six days or six months since we've spoken, we don't miss a beat. There are some I cut a lot of slack because I know the chaotic lives they lead. I am the first to put effort into a friendship, but if it is not reciprocated, eventually it will wither. There were times I was all in only later to realize it was much more valuable in my eyes than in theirs. When this happens, I have learned to move on rather than try to force something that is not worth it to the other person. If at some point, they reach out, I am likely to engage. I don't hold a grudge if I was not at the top of their priority list. I think women especially can find friendships difficult to navigate because there often ends up being some level of competition or jealousy. I do think we should challenge each other but in a kind, loving, and supportive way. Surround yourself with those who will lift you up when you are down, but who will tell it to you straight when you might need a shake-up. Forgive friends who may have hurt you and ask for forgiveness if you have caused pain. If it truly is not worth your time and energy, let it go, and be OK if someone has decided the same for you. I dedicate this chapter to every friend who has played a role in my life, no matter how big or small, how recent or distant. There are lessons to be learned from every friendship—sometimes you are the teacher and sometimes the student. No matter which end I am on, I know the outcome will be a Better Being.

Chapter Six

MIND MATTERS—
THE POWER OF THOUGHTS

HAS ANYONE EVER TOLD YOU it's all in your head? I wish I had bought into that sooner rather than later, but my appreciation for the power of the mind has been a gradual process. I have to admit I had a real attitude problem at certain times in my life, and I really wasn't sure where it was coming from. When I finally made the connection that attitude is affected by an alignment with goals and values, a lot began to make sense. I think about my experience as a gymnast, which I would say was mostly positive. I wasn't great, but I loved it. I had little natural talent or ability and often had to work twice as hard as other girls to be half as good. Learning new tricks and the sense of accomplishment that came with mastering a skill was fun and fulfilling. I never wanted to let my coaches down and tried my hardest to earn their approval. The day I showed up for the first practice after making the cut might be where some of my personal narrative began. Our coaches were a husband and wife duo, the Hardts. Phyllis went down the line, telling each girl what potential they saw and the areas where she would need to work hard to improve. When she got to me, she said, "Now, Shelley . . . Dale didn't even think you should be here, but I said, 'Oh no, that girl's got grit. She has the passion and the joy; she'll just need to work really hard.'" I know she didn't mean to make me feel bad by saying Dale didn't want me, but that was all my eight-year-old ears heard. I wasn't good and probably never would be.

Nevertheless, there I was and I was now determined to prove him wrong. It wasn't long before I elevated my skills and was ready to be on the competitive team. This was exciting but also a bit terrifying. Being in the spotlight and getting judged and ranked against other gymnasts was very uncomfortable for me. I was great in practice but often did not do well in competition. I doubted my ability, lacked confidence, and became pouty. In fact, for many years my nickname was Mona. It was kind of funny and said jokingly, but honestly, the reason I earned that nickname is nothing to brag about. My performance followed my attitude and vice versa. As one tanked so did the other. So, too, did the reactions from my coaches. I get it—it is frustrating to see someone work hard and do well in practice only to flop under pressure. Coaches have a personal investment in their gymnasts, and our performance is somewhat of a reflection on them as coaches. At least, this is the perception.

There were many occasions where I did perform well, and I'll admit winning is nice. I wish I could go back in time and watch from an external point of view to see what the difference was. Did I let my troubles with friends or difficulty with schoolwork affect my attitude and confidence, which then spilled over into the gym? The times when I was doing well, was I in a good place with schoolwork, my parents, and other influences, which led me to feel good about myself in general? Was there a certain energy in the gym—from teammates, coaches, or other athletes around—that affected my performance? I can never be sure, but knowing what I know now, my guess is yes. I think it is likely that any and all of these things were occurring and impacting my beliefs, my attitude, and my energy. One thing that is absolutely crystal clear to me today is the competition factor. I am not a competitive person by nature and although "winning" is fun, it really isn't that important to me. Understanding now that competition and winning are not priorities and values of mine, it is obvious why I struggled. I know for a fact my attitude was different during our off-season, when learning new skills and working on conditioning were the focus. I found it challenging yet fun, and it was all very motivating. I couldn't wait to get to practice during these times, but as fall neared and we began to gear up for the competitive season, the negativity crept in.

Although some respond well to the tough-love, negative-reinforcement style of coaching, I was not one of them. Phyll and Dale took turns playing good cop-bad cop, and I had a hard time managing my emotions in the face of wanting to make everyone happy. I can only imagine how difficult it is for coaches, teachers, and parents to effectively communicate minute to minute with a variety of people who have a variety of traits. I appreciate their sacrifices and the effort they invested in me to help me reach my potential. By fall of my senior year of high school, I decided I was ready to be done. I attempted to quit a few years prior, but my coaches and parents talked me out of it. This time, I knew I had to do it without warning. I was actually in a good place with both Phyll and Dale, but I had injured my knee a few months earlier, and I just didn't have the oomph to do all the hard work necessary to get ready for competition. I was afraid ending on a bad competitive season would leave a sour taste in my mouth about my whole nine-year gymnastic career, and since I knew I was not going to do college gymnastics, I decided I'd like to end while I loved the sport. My parents were shocked and not too pleased, but I am very proud that I made that big-girl decision. I am happy to say, when I showed my face a few weeks later at an exhibition performance, I was greeted with hugs and smiles. I have stayed in touch with Phyll and Dale over the years and always love getting together with them when they visit Denver. There were times in my youth when I spent more time with them than my own parents, and I am grateful for my experience. You rarely know in the moment what lessons you are learning, but there is no doubt those nine years had significant impact on my growth as a Better Being.

SELF-TALK

Do you pay attention to your self-talk? What does it sound like? If you are like most people, it is probably negative, often incorrect, and sometimes completely irrational. Where does our internal dialogue come from? Most likely it is a combination of events—personal experiences, a belief that was instilled by someone, a judgment, or a comparison. Regardless of where it began, it is important to be aware of it then do something about it! Challenge the thought. If it is negative, incorrect, or irrational, you get to decide what route to take to change course. If it IS correct, there is a major opportunity for growth. If you realize you don't like this negative talk, but it's accurate, determine what change needs to occur for it to no longer be true.

Thoughts Feelings Energy Actions

We are aware of only a small fraction of our thoughts, and although we can't keep them from entering our minds, we do get to choose what to do with them. Reflect on a time when you had a negative thought about a certain situation. How did that thought make you feel? Irritated, frustrated, or angry? Sad, lonely, worthless? The thing is, negativity is normal and serves to protect or defend us. We are wired for it, as it used to be necessary for survival. Back in the day there was no benefit to recognizing the beautiful flowers, but if we did not have the ability to detect danger, we would have been wiped out rather quickly. A big beast bearing down on us ready to chomp was not a wonderful thing, so our survival instinct—react quickly, block out other distractions, and run like hell—led us to safety. In many cases today, our perceived threats still trigger the natural inclination to defend ourselves then our minds prepare for the fight. Not only are these mechanisms not necessary for our survival, but they often prevent us from seeing options and end up holding us back.

Negative feelings are energy suckers, leaving us lethargic, drained, deflated, and apathetic. There is little desire or motivation to take action—at least not healthy action. Let's walk through an example to illustrate. Perhaps some of you will relate.

Imagine you had planned on rising early to get in a morning workout. When the alarm goes off, you hit snooze, all the while telling yourself you really should get up. After a few minutes go by, your resolve wanes. Eventually you reset the alarm for thirty minutes later and roll over. You've told yourself you will hit the gym after work, so this sleep-in won't matter, but by the time you get up and moving, the mental flogging has begun. "I am so lazy. Why am I such a loser? I am never going to lose weight because I can't seem to motivate myself to exercise." Making sure to grab your gym bag, you head to work but are a bit scrambled in the head, feeling guilty about missing your workout. When you arrive, you are greeted with a delicious treat sitting on your desk. Your coworker baked over the weekend and wanted to share the goods. Because you rushed out of the house without grabbing food, you dig right in and are instantly happy with the party going on in your mouth. A few minutes later you once again beat yourself up for not having the willpower to save it for later or to just say no, thank you. Your busy day passes by with little time for a break, and by afternoon you are tired and hungry! You wander into the break room to see if there are any leftovers from the lunch meeting earlier in the day and find all kinds of tasty morsels. Well, why not, you think: I've already blown it, so I might as well enjoy what's here. The day is finally wrapping up and you are really trying to convince yourself to get to the gym. Your bag is sitting on the passenger seat screaming at you to go, but you are tired and have so many other things to do, so you pass the exit and head on home. On your route is your favorite ice cream shop, and you decide because you are a loser and can't seem to do anything right, you might as well finish the night with something that makes you feel good. And so the cycle continues.

If you have never had any experience resembling that, you are a rare being. Most of us, in a variety of situations, have gone through this process. Negative thoughts invoke negative feelings, which generate negative energy, which leads us to negative actions. It is normal to feel bad when we don't follow through on something we had committed to doing, but the negativity that comes afterward is a choice. You have the choice to let the natural response take you into the deep, dark pit OR to challenge the thought and steer the feeling, energy, and action in a different direction.

Rewrite the Script

When you are aware of the negative conversation going on in your head, the healthy choice is to change course. Think of a time when you were in a good place mentally and emotionally. How does your posture, your attitude, and your behavior differ from when you are feeling like a dark cloud is always overhead? We stand taller with our heads up, looking around and engaging with people. We are open to possibilities and ideas. Being positive allows for the development of skills and recognition of opportunities. We've all heard the phrase, "Fake it 'til you make it," and this means you may sometimes need to tell yourself things you don't necessarily believe. Why is positive self-talk so important? Because the body responds to what the mind says.

We know that negativity is tied to the fight-orflight response, triggering a host of chemical reactions throughout the body and brain. I go into great detail on this in Chapter Seven, so for now I ask that you trust me on this! A similar yet completely opposite response occurs when we have positive thoughts. Because your brain cannot be in two places at the same time, if you swap out negative and insert positive, not only are you preventing the release of cortisol (the main player in fight or flight), but you are prompting the release of serotonin and dopamine— brain chemicals that literally make us feel good! When you feel good, you do good, and the more positive internal dialogue you engage in, the more positive the outcome will be.

Redirecting thought is very difficult (DUH! The healthy choice is the hard choice!), but it is a skill we can teach ourselves. Even people who would say they are "positive" have had to go through a process to get there. You wouldn't have to "be positive," if there were no negativity first. The rest of this chapter is devoted to practical steps you can take to enhance your skills, improve your outlook, and affect your outcomes. I have been working on them all and NONE are easy. This is where the stories get a bit tricky to tell, but so many of them played critical roles in the most recent stage of my growth, so I will do my best to keep them relevant. The last few months of my marriage, through the divorce, and well after it was final, were some very mentally challenging years for me. Disbelief, confusion, frustration, anger, resentment, and irritation were ever-present—and not just toward Travis. I will be introducing a few new characters who, ultimately, were pivotal for getting me to where I am now. Some have no idea of the impact they had, and I believe they were in my life for that fleeting moment in time for exactly this purpose—to allow me to be a Better Being. Before I dive into these concepts, I want to pick up my story where I left off in Chapter Five.

MOVING ON

Once the divorce was in process and I knew Travis and I were done, my process for moving on was to pretend it had never happened. In fact, had you taken a snapshot of my life in August of 2007 and another one in August of 2012, it would appear as though very little went on. There was no trace of Travis, or a marriage, or a divorce. Everything I had going into it, I had coming out of it—no less and no more. The economy still wasn't great, but thanks to the values instilled by my parents, I had come through the worst relatively intact. To his credit, Travis followed through on the agreement for him to repay the money I had taken out of my savings to pay off his rather significant debt. This required us to stay connected, as I received an auto-generated email each month letting me know he had deposited money into my bank account. Although that seems like such a small thing, it really annoyed me every month to receive any communication at all regarding him. I could not wait for the day the debt was paid off and there would be NO REASON ever for him to contact me again!

On the outside nothing had changed, but the essence of who I was definitely had. Gone was that fun, funny, confident girl who was open and trusting and kind. In her place was a girl filled with doubt, who believed very little of what anyone told her. I found myself watching strangers and wondering what secrets they were keeping from their significant others, or what bomb that woman was going to drop on her husband tonight. I saw a lie embedded in every sentence and questioned my own judgment and ability to make a good decision. I was cynical and skeptical of everyone and everything. I actually kept most of this to myself, but my brain was busy with these thoughts and the scenarios I pondered. I was closed off, kept my head down, and had no desire to interact with anyone other than my very close circle.

One occasion when I did interact was with a group of people I knew through Cigna. We had all participated in an event for the

American Heart Association and were socializing afterward. A conversation with one person in particular started to get personal, and when he asked me about my status, the words got stuck in my throat. I never considered how disgusting it would feel to say, "I'm divorced." It was an experience I was not prepared for and left me feeling physically sick. He'd been part of Cigna for only a short time and had no idea about any of my past, but he was the first person outside my immediate circle I said the words out loud to. The flood of emotion that came with it was unexpected and a little embarrassing, and I am forever grateful that his reaction was kind and sincere. Interestingly enough, this same person had played a huge role the previous year, a role he was completely unaware of. I happened to be walking into the Cigna offices to give their team a training on stress management when I opened one of the difficult emails from Travis. Having just read this, I knew it was going to be tough to compose myself to get through the class, and I needed a distraction to focus on—especially given the topic! I always felt welcomed by the Denver Cigna team, and there was a new addition who was young, cute, and lighthearted. It was exactly the distraction I needed from the heaviness I had just read and felt. There was good-natured ribbing going on by all parties, and the new guy took it all in stride. I honestly cannot imagine how I would have held up had he not been there and been such a good sport. Our paths have crossed very few times since, but it is a perfect example of why I believe every person enters our world for a reason. I appreciate him having entered mine to ease the blow of two difficult situations.

After finally saying "I'm divorced" out loud, the anger toward Travis welled up to new levels. It was his fault I even had to say those words and be in these uncomfortable situations. I had no desire to experience that again so I decided to move along through life as a single gal, with no intention of having any kind of real relationship again. Why bother—people are only going to let you down in the end anyway. I'm sure these are common thoughts and feelings for someone who has gone through a significant breakup, but feeling this way was foreign to me and I truly did not feel like myself. Even though my relationship with David ended in a rather explosive fashion, I had not had anywhere close to this reaction. To me the clear difference was not only that Travis and I were married (vs. engaged to David) but also the level of connection that was shared was different. Travis and I absolutely operate on the same frequency and were very in tune with each other's energy. I was so angry at him for tuning us out that I decided it was best to shut everything down. He snuffed out my spirit, and I would just have to get through life on my own.

In some ways this served me quite well. I focused all my energy on my business, my close friends and family, and my self-care. One major move I knew I needed to make was to get out of my condo, which I had lived in since 2003. Travis and I lived there together, and I really felt like a change of scenery was necessary. Back in 2006 a new high-rise had been built on the other side of town, and I had always wanted to live there. It was the epitome of luxury living and highly coveted. I knew the chances of getting in were slim, but I kept my eyes peeled for anything to come available. In June of 2013 my wishes came true. By this time in Denver, the real estate market was getting out of control, but through sheer will, I signed the lease, found tenants to move into my condo, moved, and went on a trip to London—all in the span of two weeks. I had been a property owner since the age of twenty-six, so to now be a renter at nearly forty-one was unsettling to me, but my feet were in the door of my dreams, and I knew it would all work out. I loved the new environment and the chance to create a completely new space. The only residual energy from my past came in the form of our cats, Bode and Axle. There is no way I would ever give them up, so the three of us would just have to figure it out!

Life was pretty good. It was fun to explore a different side of town, and I slowly was beginning to interact with my new neighbors. By fall of that year Travis had paid off all his debt, and cutting that final tie was a milestone I'd been waiting for. He had done a few things along the way that I know were his attempt to start a conversation. I never took the bait and was hopeful that now there would be no more bait thrown my way! As I mentioned in Chapter Five, my motto for the new year was to not be so lame. I was feeling better in a lot of ways and was ready to start having fun again. My professional life was at its peak thus far, the finances were healthy, I weathered some awful storms (literally!) regarding my rental properties, and it truly felt like I was making a comeback. There was even a man in the mix! Nothing serious at all—just someone I was noticing at the gym and was pretty sure he was noticing me. I proceeded very cautiously, but it was obvious we were mutually interested, and each time we were at the gym, we got to know a little more about the other. Then in August of that year, a major swirl of energy roughed up my world.

By this time Brian (the gym guy) and I had been chatting for about six weeks. We never exchanged numbers or last names, but at the gym we were spending more time talking than working out. I found it curious that he had not asked me out, but I chalked it up to him just ending a relationship or being in the process and not ready to step out quite yet. He knew I was divorced and was probing about my history, but I told him it was way too much of a story for the gym. I had also decided I was going to reveal myself at a much slower pace than I had in the past because, really, what's the rush? One day at the gym I glanced in the mirror and saw a familiar face—more specifically, a familiar smile. You met Brandon last chapter—my friend who has a unique concept of time—but Brandon and I had not seen each other in years. When he caught my reflection, he turned around and picked me up in the biggest bear hug. You'd have thought he just learned he won the lottery by the joy and excitement he was expressing. I am not elevating myself to any kind of status—this is just Brandon. He is a force of positive energy that is infectious and entirely genuine. He is the kind of person who lights up every space he enters and leaves you feeling better than you started. No. Matter. What. For any of this to make sense, I need to fill in the backstory.

Brandon first came into my life about two years before I met Travis. He was a very green trainer, and I kind of took him under my wing to help him develop and reach his potential in the industry. I knew this guy could change lives—he just had to focus and channel his energy in the right way. We spent a lot of time working out, riding bikes, talking about business, and partaking in our favorite activity—eating. He is a miracle story, having survived a horrific motorcycle accident two years prior to my meeting him. Brandon is walking proof of the resilience of the human body, and his mission is to spread this message and empower people to believe in it for themselves. He is a bundle of love and light, and he shares it with everyone. I loved Brandon in so many ways, but in other ways he drove me batshit crazy! One of the things that drove me crazy was how ridiculously positive he always was. Ugh, seriously! Not everything is great and wonderful, but Brandon will try to make you think so. If I was complaining about something, he always had a positive spin on it. I did not understand where all this positive energy came from and, quite honestly, I often tried to squash it. Being the imposing six-feet and 185 pounds of shredded mass that he is, I was never successful. He was positive. No. Matter. What. And it did start to rub off. At the time I am sure I was not fully aware of the concept of the transfer of energy, but I think Brandon was in my life to open me up to positive energy—both giving and receiving it.

Due to life circumstances we started spending less time together and shortly after I met Travis. Given how magical that was at the time, I felt Brandon's energy ignited my energy and opened up space for love and the incredible connection with Travis to settle in. Sadly, I eliminated Brandon from my life a few months later. He had left me a message early in the morning on my birthday in November—a very kind, warm, energetic, PLATONIC message. Travis was having none of it. He lost his mind that a guy "from my past" would be calling me to wish me a happy birthday at 6:30 a.m. Travis had met Brandon and knew that we had been friends for a few years, so I was totally taken aback by this reaction. By that time, we were living together, well on our way to getting engaged and married. I certainly didn't want there to be any doubt or question in his mind about my relationship with Brandon, so I decided it was best to cut ties. As I was driving to train a client later that morning, I called Brandon and told him the news. I was bawling. It was awful to tell someone you really love and care about on a human level, who has been nothing but good to you, that you can't talk to them anymore. He didn't understand it but honored my request. It is one of my very few regrets in life, and when I saw Brandon at the gym nearly seven years later, I knew he had reentered my life for a reason. At that moment it wasn't clear, but the events that were to unfold over the next year left no doubt. It was about to get really ugly, and I was going to need as much positive energy around me as possible.

Next up is an interesting, crazy ride that revved up with a confluence of events. Event one was seeing Brandon in the gym and knowing we would reconnect as friends. Events two and three are dreams that happened one week apart. I had the first one the evening of Sunday, August 10, and it went like this:

> *I am sobbing and my mind is reeling through snippets of my life with Travis. I keep saying, "his poor heart, his poor heart." His stepmom, Marsha, is there, and she is telling me there was nothing they could do for him. My whole life with Travis is racing through my brain as I continue to sob uncontrollably, repeating "his poor heart."*

When I woke up, Bode and Axle were sitting on me looking very alarmed. I was crying out loud, and my pillow was soaking wet. I couldn't stop crying, and I knew in my soul that something had happened with Travis. I had to share this with someone, so I immediately called Lisa, my BFF of more than twenty years, and told her my dream. I didn't know what to do with it and I was extremely shaken. Later that day (the eleventh) the news of Robin Williams's suicide came out. He was one of Travis's favorite actors, and I knew whenever there was news of suicide or someone with bipolar disorder, Travis was deeply affected. At this time, I didn't know how to interpret anything, but I knew there had been a major shift in his energy. I knew it, because I felt it.

Later that week, I saw Brian at the gym, and our usual banter took place. I held back my temptation to ask if he wanted to grab coffee or something to meet up outside of the gym. I was committed to waiting for him to take this further, but it was starting to bug me that he was clearly interested but hadn't asked me out! That weekend I had a dream that gave me my answer.

I am out with friends and the place looks like a nightclub version of The Cheesecake Factory. Through the crowd, I see Brian and point him out to my friends. He sees me, and I am about to walk over to him when I see an almost imperceptible shake of his head. I realize he is telling me not to come over because his wife is with him.

When I woke up, I knew that was the answer. He was married. I planned to call him out on that the next time I saw him at the gym. That opportunity came almost a week later, and, as per usual, we gravitated toward each other while working out and got into a conversation. He once again steered the conversation, trying to get me to open up about my marriage and divorce, but I shut it down. I then asked, "What about you? What's your story? Let me guess . . . wife and kids waiting for you at home?"

His silence and the look on his face said it all. I actually was dumbfounded—couldn't believe it. How was this guy, who wore no ring and presented himself as unattached, married!?! I believe my actual words were, "you motherfucker." Of course he had an explanation—"It's not what you think . . . it's a loveless marriage . . .we live in separate wings of the house." Blah. Blah. Blah. The story was, he had been married for thirteen years, with two kids, ages two and six. Early on in their marriage he had had a pretty good drug addiction, which she helped him overcome. He had now been clean for eight years and once he got sober, he realized he actually didn't like her. He thought she was a pretty awful person and before their youngest was born, they separated twice. His claim was he felt obligated to stay together for the kids and because of all the bs she put up with from him. I was so disgusted by what I was hearing that I just walked away. I couldn't believe that A) my dream was accurate and B) that I finally opened myself up to possibility, only to have the reality of what is really out there show itself. For the next two weeks, I ignored him, refusing to make eye contact and walking the other direction when I saw him coming my way.

I was really unnerved by these three things happening all at once—Brandon reappearing, the dream about Travis, and the realization that Brian was married. I didn't know at the time what any of it meant, why it was happening, and why all the events occurred at the same time. Each on its own was noteworthy, but together, I felt there was great significance. The life lesson I was to learn ended up taking approximately a full year.

My reaction to the discovery of Brian being married may seem a bit much to some of you. After all, we never went out and didn't even know each other's last names. All I can say is, you weren't there for the conversations. Brian and I had a very real connection—one that he readily acknowledged. I felt like I had been lied to and cheated on, and my heightened sensitivity due to the Travis dream really set me back. After a few weeks of the silent treatment, Brian approached me and I had no escape. He stood in front of me for forty-five minutes and apologized. He said it was killing him to have me ignore him and to see me completely shut down. He had no idea our friendly interactions were going to lead to feelings, and he knew he had to tell me somehow but just didn't know how to bring it up. He said he felt like he had lost a best friend and asked for my forgiveness. Blah. Blah. Blah. Although I applauded his effort, tail between the legs and all, I wasn't sure he deserved my forgiveness. I said very little at that time, other than to point out all the logical opportunities he had had to mention a wife and kids. He had obliterated the opportunity for us to be friends, and all I now saw was another guy who says what he needs to say in the moment to have an outcome he wants. I was angry for so many reasons but few had to do with the fact that he was unavailable. In my opinion there was no need for this "friendship" to ever have started, and I planned on shutting him out.

I need to fast-forward through a lot of what took place in the months that followed or this chapter will never end. In summary I eventually came around. Being angry takes a lot of effort, and the truth is I didn't like it. I am not an angry person, so it required a lot of work for me to pull it off. Brian and I resumed our connection, with me working hard to stay firmly in the friend zone. He loved to push boundaries, but I didn't budge. I still refused to share much of my story with him, and we never exchanged numbers or last names. Quite honestly, I didn't trust either of us if we had a way of getting in touch outside of the gym. We went through a few tugging matches over the next nine months, with me disappearing for weeks at a time simply because I didn't have the bandwidth to deal with him on top of all the other energy swirling about.

From August through Thanksgiving, the Travis dreams were relentless. These also made me angry, as did an email I received in September. This was another "apology" email from him and was the most pathetic one yet. Knowing him as I did, I suspected that he was in the beginning of a new relationship and, because he knew I hated him, he couldn't focus on the new girl. He needed to do something, anything, to, hopefully, get me to respond so he could work his Travis charm and eventually win me over. He could then move forward with who was next. I ignored the email and the dreams kept coming. One dream right around my birthday was particularly difficult for me.

We are riding the Harley (something we did quite often in real life), and obviously there has been an accident. I am lying on the side of the road, and he is standing over me but is fading away like a hologram disappearing. I am reaching out my hand, crying, saying, "Please don't leave me," and he is crying and saying, "I'm sorry I didn't protect you." We are both repeating these words and eventually he is completely gone.

Our final therapy session was just a few days after my birthday. I am pretty sure my grand exit was forever burned in his memory, which is probably why I felt his energy this time. My lack of response to his email was, no doubt, eating at him. The sound of silence tended to do that! My mind was so full from the dreams, analyzing them then being pissed off about them, that I had little energy for other noise. I stayed away from my gym through the new year and had decided when I went back, I would not interact with Brian. The feelings were still there, and it was just getting to be too much. Funny enough, he had also started showing up in my dreams, and there were several where he and Travis morphed into one another. Hey, I told you in the beginning to buckle up for this chapter. If you find it crazy reading this, think of what I was going through living it!

I knew I needed to do something to shut off the connection with Travis if I ever was to get back to living my life. I could determine what I chose to think about when I was awake, but the intrusion during sleep was beyond my control. I went to an intuitive therapist, Fran Gallaher, who helps people break through mental and emotional blocks through a variety of techniques. Once she got my backstory, she suggested I work on a few things. One, I had to stop pretending my life with Travis did not exist. Two, I should acknowledge and embrace that what we had was real, was special, and was rare. And three, I would need to forgive him and myself. Good god, really? UGH. This was going to be hard. And yet, I knew it needed to be done if I really wanted to move forward. She asked me to write each day, thirty positive things currently happening in my life. I also was to write things I loved about my life with Travis, as well as the specific things I would need to forgive. She also suggested I remain open to Brian, not in a romantic way but on a human level. Her feeling was he was playing an important role that might be different from what either one of us initially thought, so I should follow it to the end. I was not thrilled about any of her recommendations, but I took them under advisement.

The most significant breakthrough came at a later session when she took me on a guided meditation. Before we began, Fran told me she would be walking me along a beautiful path, eventually reaching the "temple of my soul." When I got there, a guardian angel would escort me to a magnificent room where I would wait for people who were destined to appear so I could speak to them. She instructed me to simply be part of the journey, not to try to make anyone show up but to just let what would be, be. When someone presented themselves, I could say whatever I felt needed to be said. Her one caveat was that if Travis did not appear on his own, I must call for him. I had no idea what to expect, but I got comfortable, settled in, and followed along as she led me on this adventure into a great unknown. I had dabbled with hypnosis before, but this was nothing like that. I could feel myself becoming weightless yet still fully aware of what was happening around me. The image of the path was a gorgeous, somewhat secret hike I had done a few times in Hawaii—at the time known only to locals. When I arrived at the temple of my soul, my guardian angel was a former client of mine, Rosemary Brown. Rosemary was an absolutely incredible woman who I had known for a relatively brief time. She had been in a battle with ovarian cancer for twenty years, and I was seeing her twice a week at her house to help improve her strength and balance. She didn't know me when I was with David but was there from the start with Travis. Rosemary was so happy for us to have found this love and even hosted an engagement party for us. She passed away in the spring of 2011, and her memorial gathering was incredibly moving. It was very intimate, as all who attended had been personally invited by her husband, Bill. I felt a bit out of place because most of the people had known Rosemary for many years, and as we sat in a circle, Bill proceeded to tell what we each meant to her. Travis attended this with me, and when Bill got to us, I was overcome with emotion. I had no idea how much my twice-weekly visits meant to her and how much joy she experienced through my joy. We often had indepth conversations about life and relationships and love—both finding and losing it. Rosemary was the epitome of strength and grace. She had no problem telling me if I was off-base and on many occasions opened me to seeing things from a different perspective. My time with her absolutely made me a Better Being so it came as no surprise when she appeared as my guardian angel for this important part of my growth.

Fran continued to describe the room where I would wait, and as Rosemary faded away, Fran became silent. It wasn't long before the first person appeared—Dale, my gymnastics coach. I saw myself forgiving him for not wanting me because I wasn't going to be good enough to be on the team. During all my years in gymnastics and through numerous subsequent visits, I had never spoken of this. I clearly held tight to the sentiment, offering another example of feeling like I don't belong, but it was time to let it go. Next up, my grandfather. I gave a bit of history in the previous chapter, but let me just say now, he was a harsh man. Visiting my grandparents was not something I ever looked forward to. After I quit gymnastics, in the height of my fat years, the visits became unbearable. One particular visit in my early twenties was the final straw. There was constant commentary, judgment, and criticism, and I'd had enough. My grandfather, my father, and I were sitting at the breakfast table, eating something quite normal—a bowl of cereal—when my grandfather said to me, "Should you be eating that? It seems like you don't really need it." I put my spoon down, rose from the table, and said, "Fuck you, Grandpa." I walked out the door and never spoke to him again. As he appeared during this meditation, I apologized to him and forgave him. I acknowledged that he had done the best he could with the tools he had, and I am sure in some way he thought his comments were made to help me.

As the image of my grandfather disappeared, I began having strange sensations. My whole body felt like it was swelling up, growing very large. It seemed as though my head was gigantic and my hands were enormous. At the same time, I felt completely absent from my body, both feeling my surroundings and feeling nothing at all. My throat became constricted, and I was having a hard time breathing. Tears began flooding out, but I was completely still. And there he was. Unlike with Dale and my grandfather, I did not see me—only Travis. He looked very small, but I'm not sure if that was only because I felt so uncomfortably large. In that moment all I could think was "thank you for loving me."

I am not sure how long I was in this state, but at one point Fran asked if my work was done. I nodded my head, and as she started walking me back down the path, my body slowly began to shrink. The tears stopped, breathing was easy, and I was back in her room just as we had begun. I described to Fran everything

I had experienced, and we spent a bit of time analyzing each phase. The three who appeared had all caused deep wounds, and no doubt I was carrying the hurt and anger from each situation for all these years. The damage caused by Travis was the most significant. Fran shared the insight that I had to become larger than life and very uncomfortable as a way of acknowledging that Travis loved me; this made a lot of sense. Although pretending as though our life together didn't happen and determining there was no way he could have loved me like he said he did initially allowed me to survive the storm, it had worn out its usefulness. She likened it to having a hole in your head, applying compression to stop the bleeding, then going on as if there is no hole in your head. Pretending it's not there doesn't make it so! Accepting, letting go, and forgiving are all necessary for tending to our emotional wounds. And none of those are easy. I'd love to report that after this guided meditation, I never had hurt or anger again, but that would be false. It was, however, a huge step, not only in my acknowledgment and acceptance of the connection with Travis but also in my belief that continuing to work on forgiveness was going to be necessary for me to truly move on to live my best life. The hard work was not over; more so, it had just begun.

After the new year I went back to the gym and was immediately greeted by Brian. Although I contemplated Fran's advice, I wasn't feeling up to the challenge of fostering a friendship. In my effort to cut this tie I was rather cold and short in my response. I brushed him off, and as I watched him walk away, I felt like a horrible human being. I suddenly saw a wounded little boy who just had someone tell him she no longer wanted him around. I really am not that person but felt this was the best way to protect myself. Over the next few months I did my best to avoid Brian, but he was infiltrating my dreams more frequently. I felt like he and Travis were scheming together to drive me insane—and it was working! Here is one that really messed with my head.

I am back in my high school in Winneconne, and Travis and I are in the hallway talking. He is apologizing for all the hurt he has caused, and he hands me a note. I am not really interested in what he has to say, but I take the note and start to open it. Before I read it, I look up, and he is now Brian. Brian is asking me what the note says . . . he tells me he can't help me if he doesn't know what happened.

It was after that dream that I thought perhaps Fran was right. Maybe Brian was in my life to help me break through this fortress I had built up inside my soul. It was time to tell Brian the story, and I decided the next time he was at the gym, I would start a conversation with him. It had been quite some time since we'd spoken, so I wasn't sure how I would be received, but when I approached, he did not hesitate. I was still determined not to exchange any contact information, so after a brief chat, we agreed to meet the following day in a park near my house at a designated time. I was nervous for a lot of reasons—would I get through the story without crying? Was he going to think I was a whackadoo? Was he going to push any boundaries and would I let him cross them? UGH, all of this was Travis's fault!

The next day it was odd seeing Brian in something other than gym clothes and out of our regular environment, and I think we both felt a bit awkward. After nine months of dancing around our emotions, we did share an intimate moment. It was just a kiss, which for a lot of people is no big deal, but given he was married, I am not super proud of it. At the time it seemed practically unavoidable, and once that was out of the way, I started my story. Two hours and a lot of tears later, Brian was caught up. He now knew almost every detail from when I met Travis to the present moment. It was definitely more of a story than he imagined, and he understood why I reacted to his role in this saga the way I did. It felt good to get it out and to express what

I had been going through to someone with whom I also shared a connection. After our meeting in the park Brian and I had a few conversations in the gym and, ultimately, he is the one who made me face the reality of what I needed to do. One day while on the stair-climbers, I told him about a dream I had just had.

> *I am getting ready to teach one of my classes and am putting handouts by the seating areas. There is a tall, dark figure enshrouded in a black cloak standing in a corner of the room. I say hello and ask if they are here for the class, and we have this exchange:*
>
> *"No, I just want you to be my friend."*
>
> *Me: "I have a lot of friends already and am busy getting ready to teach a class."*
>
> *"But I need you to be my friend so you can save my life."*
>
> *Me: "Oh, honey, I'm sorry but I don't do that anymore."*
>
> *At that point, the figure crumbles and ends up as a pile of black cloak on the floor.*

After I told Brian this dream, he said to me, "You know what you need to do, right? You know you need to see him and talk to him." This is the last thing I ever wanted to do, but I knew he was right. I knew the dreams would not end and the energy connection would never be broken unless I faced this in real life. I was not happy about it, but it was the answer. After that conversation, without warning, I took a six-month hiatus from that gym. Many of the conversations with Brian were getting uncomfortable, and to save us both I thought it was best to stay away. I also knew I had a daunting task ahead and would need all my energy to get through it. During that time I had plenty of dreams, all of great significance, and the resolve to finally see Travis was building. The summer of 2015 was a busy one. I was in the midst of a big remodel project at one of my rental properties and had several trips planned. I wanted to have a clear calendar before I reached out, then in July and August several signs presented that let me know it was time.

One day I had some business to do at the Cigna office in Denver. Travis happened to work in the same complex, and I was a little uneasy as I drove there, hoping that I wouldn't run into him. There are nearly five-thousand people who work in three towers, so it was unlikely, but still the thought crossed my mind. As I pulled up to the garage, a group of people were crossing the street and guess who was leading the pack?! His head was down—buried in his phone—so I knew he didn't see me, but my heart lurched and my stomach churned. He looked different—not the lanky, clean-shaven, fresh smiling face of the man I married, but one who was much heavier, with a full beard and an intensity about him. I drove past and proceeded to the farthest space possible. On my drive home I stopped for a quick errand and at one point checked my email. I had one from LinkedIn, telling me someone was looking at my profile. Of course I was curious to see who it was, and again my heart lurched and my stomach churned. WHY, why, why was Travis looking at my profile?! Had he actually seen me as I drove past? I really didn't think so, but it was too much of a coincidence. I was so irritated but did nothing about it.

I had many dreams in the following weeks, and the following one in mid-August was quite powerful. Here is a little information to help you follow: Becky is a childhood friend who is very dear to me. Travis and I attended her wedding in Wisconsin in 2009. I've owned a rental property at Lake Ozark, Missouri, since 2005, and it has been nothing but a nightmare from the get-go. Every year I have been saying I need to get rid of it; it just hasn't happened yet.

Travis and I are at what seems to be an engagement party for Becky and her fiancé, and we are having a lovely time. At one point I lose track of him, but then notice that he is off in the corner having a very intimate conversation with Becky. When I walk over, it is quite clear what I have barged in on. At this point Travis disappears, and I am livid with Becky. I cannot believe what is happening, and she is telling me he is not who I think he is and she is doing me a favor. It is all so absurd to me, but now I am in a house alone. It is dark and the house is kind of falling apart. I am sick on a couch, and Travis comes over to take care of me. He is super tall, as if he is on stilts, and has really baggy jeans that have to be held up with suspenders. He is drowning in these clothes. He keeps trying to comfort me, and I tell him he needs to leave, that he needs to go and never come back. I tell him as soon as I feel better I will be selling this house, and he asks if I need a ride to the airport. I tell him no, that I don't need his help. I've always done everything myself, and I can find my own way to the Springfield airport. His departure is very sad for both of us, but he finally leaves. The house now becomes bright, and I am no longer sick. Becky is there. I'm not mad at her and tell her to go be with him. He will need someone to take care of him—it is no longer my role.

If I wasn't clear on what I needed to do, that very day sealed the deal. I was driving down Speer Boulevard, a main drag in Denver. As I pulled up to a red light, I glanced at the vehicle to my left—a green truck. My heart lurched and my stomach churned. It was Travis. With all my heart and soul, I could have sworn it was him. But it was the Travis I knew—clean-shaven, wearing a T-shirt with the sleeves cut out and a hat on backward. It was even a hat I had given him, a sort of vintage-looking Boston Red Sox hat. He looked my way and I immediately turned.

We played this game of looking and turning away a few times. I wasn't sure if it was him—could he have lost this much weight in the last five weeks? With Travis, it's totally possible! The one sure marker—a sleeve tattoo on his left arm—was out of my view, and as the light changed, I drove straight, and he made a left turn. I was a little freaked out. Was it him or did I manifest that vision? It didn't really matter at this point—I knew I had to reach out to see if he would meet with me. And so, eleven months and two days after receiving his apology email, I finally responded. The following is the actual email exchange:

August 14, 2015

It has been nearly a year since you sent me your apology email. I can't really describe the rush of emotion that went through me when I read it. None of it good, which is why I never responded . . . . still protecting you after all these years. Your email was actually the 3rd of a trio of events that happened within days of each other and set into motion a path I needed to go down.

You'd think that after almost four years of not speaking to you I'd be just fine. The unfinished business and lack of closure has definitely affected me. The problem is even though I haven't spoken to you, there has still been contact. I'm not just talking about the times you've reached out, but in other ways that are too hard to explain over email.

I came to a conclusion a few months ago and it is one I was really hoping to avoid. My strategy of trying to move forward as if you never existed has reached the ceiling. In many ways my life is amazing. That's because I've buried my head and worked my ass off. It's a great distraction with nice outcomes but doesn't solve everything. In a big way my life is not amazing, and I know it never has a chance to be unless I do something.

I have been waiting for the right time to send this, when I'll be strong enough to deal with everything, but I don't think there ever will be a right time. My dreams have been more frequent and more intense and I'm pretty sure I saw you yesterday—I'm taking that as a sign that I can't put this off any longer.

I am writing this to ask if you'd be willing to meet with me to see if I can finally put all that is going on to rest. I don't know when or where or even how it's all going to look. If you'll meet me, we can take our time figuring all that out.

Michelle

Travis

My apology email was terrible. I've gone back and read it multiple times since then and I realize it fell well short. Yes, I would be more than willing to meet with you. I know this email is short. I'm filled with a rush of emotion right now and I don't want to say the wrong thing over email. Not that I have anything negative to say to you. I just don't want to screw up this opportunity to meet.

Me

OK, I think we both need to let this sit. I don't want to get into an email conversation. I am heading out of town for the weekend. I can email you when I get back to figure it out.

I just need to know one thing now—were you driving down Speer around 3 yesterday? I was at a stoplight next to someone and it was you—the you I remember, even down to a Red Sox hat. The only reason I'm questioning it is because you were in a green Tundra, and the Travis I know would not be driving a green truck. But I couldn't shake that it was you—and you looked at me several times as if to decide if it was me you were seeing.

Travis

OK, letting it sit sounds just fine. Nope, I was not on Speer yesterday nor do I drive a green truck.

I look forward to your email when you're back. Have a good weekend.

THE MEETING

We planned to meet the following weekend on neutral territory. Cheesman Park at 1 o'clock on Saturday. I arrived early . . . and so did he. As I was walking from my car to a bench to wait, I saw him heading my way. Within seconds all my hate and anger washed away. I'm not sure how or why, but I felt nothing but sadness and compassion for the person walking toward me. I knew immediately that he was in a really awful place, and I naturally reverted to only wanting him to be OK. It was a hesitant, nervous greeting and eventually we made our way to a spot and settled in. He began by saying that I should ask him anything and everything, and he promised to be 100 percent truthful. I promised the same, then there was a long, painful silence. I knew what I needed to ask but didn't really know how to begin—and I was afraid of being right. The silence was too much and he started to speak, but I jumped in and said, "Last summer around August, something was happening. I don't know what, but there was a major energy shift and it hasn't let up." He immediately started to cry and began to tell me something, but I stopped him. I needed to get it out before he told me anything. "I had a dream," I said, "a really awful dream, and I think I know what it means." He was now crying uncontrollably and asked, "Was it about suicide?" At that, I lost it. It was the answer I was afraid of, not only because he was going through a difficult time, but because I KNEW he was going through it. It confirmed for me that I am connected to him in a way that is not normal, and I am very sensitive to his energy. I had no doubt that all the dreams I had over the past year were telling me what was happening in his life. I wasn't sure how to feel about this. I was definitely not happy because I didn't want to be connected to someone who caused me so much pain. I would much rather have been wrong, so I could chalk up my dreams to an overactive imagination.

But I wasn't wrong. For the next eight hours we talked, and laughed, and cried. I told him all the dreams I had, and he confirmed things that he had gone through. The first dream I had coincided with him being at his lowest point that led to his closest brush with suicide. His apology email came in September, then the dreams were relentless. I asked if he had started seeing someone around that time, and he said yes. Her name was Emily and he met her shortly after this incident. He said she was compassionate and patient, and in those ways she reminded him of me. I pressed him—there was something else about her that connected us. He then told me she was from Wisconsin and was a huge Packers fan. Well, that explained a lot. Travis and I used to watch every Packers game together. I am an avid fan, and he was totally on board and became one too. He admitted that every time they watched the games, he was thinking of me. I know! I was having dreams several times a week at that time. Sometime later I saw a picture of Emily—turns out she resembles my friend Becky. When I told him about the Harley accident dream, he said he always thinks about me around my birthday and is especially sorry for how he treated me the last one, right before our final therapy appointment.

At times in our meeting, it was as if the last four years had not happened. We were just Travis and Michelle having a day together. At other times, I was overwhelmed with emotion of all that had happened and I didn't hold back. I told him everything about Brandon and how my ending our friendship was one of my deepest regrets. He couldn't believe I had not met anyone and was still single, but once I detailed how I not only had no trust in men, I had no trust in myself to be a good judge of character, he got it. I told him about Brian and how that set me back again, but in the end, it was because of him that I was even here today. Travis told me the last four years had been awful for him and that leaving me was a huge mistake. He said he told everyone he knows that I was the most amazing wife a man could ask for, and he would never find this kind of love again. If he could go back, he would do it all differently. He ended up dating Kendall for a little over a year and eventually found her cheating on him, and he figured he deserved it for how he treated me. He said he can't believe the life we had and the one he walked away from, but he wasn't in his right mind. I reminded him that I kept telling him that, and he said at that point I was the enemy. It made no sense to him either, but I was the thing he needed to get away from. He was sorry for everything and has spent the last four years beating himself up for the damage he caused. It was obvious he has not been living a healthy lifestyle, but he said he was working on that. He said Emily helps with that as she is pretty healthy, and I asked if she knows him. Like really knows him. "Only as much as I let her. Nobody will ever know me like you do" was his reply.

We grabbed a bite to eat, and at one point we both looked up at the same time knowing exactly what the other was thinking. What was this? A final day for closure and goodbye? The beginning of mending, healing, and new possibility? I went into this day with no expectations and was going to end it with no expectations. He went into this day expecting a beatdown, feeling guilty but relieved that he didn't receive one. I told him I forgave him and asked that he forgive himself. There was no need for further punishment—everyone had suffered enough. Eventually Travis got a text from Emily asking what was taking so long. . . . "Maybe you are having too good a time with your ex-wife?" It was time to part ways, but neither of us knew how to end it. Eventually we hugged and cried and said our goodbyes, each of us committing to doing what felt right, whatever that looked like.

As I walked away, I knew I would never get back together with Travis. I felt free. I was relieved to have had the opportunity to have a final say, get my questions answered, and validate my feelings. I knew he did me a huge favor by leaving me. He is not well and has a very difficult life ahead of him. Events unfolded in the following weeks that truly provided the perfect ending for my other (yet unwritten) book. There are way too many details to go into, but let's just say, the master manipulator nearly duped me again. I caught on and, unfortunately for him, put a little snag in his plan. It was no longer my job to make Travis's life easier for him. He could and would figure it out, and I wished him all the best. I hope to never hear from him again, but I won't be surprised if I do.

I have worked hard to deflect his energy when it comes my way. A trip in September of 2016 to my favorite psychic in Aspen tuned me into this. I was still having dreams and was irritated with these intrusions. I didn't understand why I had to be the chosen one! I had forgiven and let go and truly was OK with how everything turned out, so why was I still so connected to him? I had not mentioned anything about my relationship with Travis, but at one point the psychic said, "There is someone from your past who is bothering you. He has moved on and you don't see him, but he's still part of you and you don't like it." WOW! I told her yes, I have dreams about my ex-husband and have always been sensitive to his energy. I asked why I still have the connection—shouldn't his new girlfriend or wife or whatever he has be the one who has the connection? She laughed and said, "Oh no dear, it doesn't work that way. You were together in a past life and in this one and will forever be connected to him. You don't get to choose." Well, that's not what I wanted to hear! Seriously, I will never be able to get rid of him? I asked how I am supposed to deal with this, and she said, "All you need to do when you feel his energy, is light it with love and send it on its way. Do not give it strength by committing your energy to it."

At the time that seemed really goofy, but I actually started doing it, and I have to say, I am a believer. You see, to resist something that is happening often makes it stronger. My negativity surrounding the dreams and my feeling his energy only made them more powerful. If I just accept what is, and be kind and loving with it, I can wish it well and send it away. If I find myself with any thoughts of Travis, I literally make a heart shape with my hands, think a happy thought (unrelated to him), and send it all off by blowing a kiss. I now practice this anytime I am around negativity, as I would rather spend that time and energy on things that matter. I have little patience for it and will do my best to divert attention or a conversation toward something positive.

POSITIVE MANTRA

Steering attention away from negativity can be quite a feat, especially when it is rolling around in your head! When we try to stop the chatter, we often end up scolding ourselves. "I need to stop thinking about that. Why can't I let that go? What is wrong with me that I can't stop replaying that?" This is the tactic we typically employ, and yet it is just more negativity! When I was going through the yuckiness of my divorce, Lisa sent me a meme that said. "Keep Your Heels, Head, and Standards High." It resonated with me and I decided to adopt this as my own personal mantra. When I find myself swimming in mud, this is the reminder that helps me crawl out of it. You can't think two things at the same time, so having a specific go-to phrase is quite effective, because it completely redirects your thought. I printed this meme, put it in a blingy frame (everything's better with bling!), and placed it on my dresser in my closet. I see it multiple times a day, and it is fully ingrained in my head. I have been practicing being positive for quite a few years now, and it really does start to come naturally. Because I have consistently steered my thoughts away from negativity, the new automatic pathway has been deeply carved, and I rarely have to use my mantra.

Whew, we made it! Yes, we! This was a tough one to write, and I'm sure a bit challenging to read. There is a lot going on in this chapter, but it all comes down to this—your thoughts are powerful! If you harness the power and steer it in the right direction, a world of possibility will open up. If you are ready to break through your mental obstacles, here are some things to consider:

1. Be aware of the negative self-talk that is holding you back. Challenge it and commit to an alternate conversation.

2. Get in tune with your thoughts, energy, and actions. Come up with your own positive mantra to help steer away from negative thoughts.

3. Incorporate a mind-body practice into your lifestyle— deep breathing, visualization, guided imagery, and meditation all provide great benefits.

4. Consider outside help to break through emotional barriers. An energy healer, intuitive therapist, or spiritual guide may offer new insights that lead to your growth.

5. Determine what your mind is full of—anger, guilt, resentment, hurt, worry. Commit to honing your skills to forgive, let go, and be present.

FINAL THOUGHTS

There are so many thoughts in this chapter, I am not sure anyone needs a final one, so I am going to keep it simple by summarizing the lessons I gleaned from some of these life experiences.

Barriers to accepting, forgiving, and letting go are some of the most difficult to overcome, but it is impossible to live your best life unless and until these are accomplished. Sometimes you think you have worked past all of it, only to be smacked in the face with it at some other time. If this happens, there is more work to be done at a deeper level. It is hard and annoying and frustrating, and you may need to attack it from a variety of angles, but it is worth it! The freedom that comes when you have truly cut an anchor is indescribable, and there is now time and energy for good things to enter your space.

People who come in and out of your life at various times may be there for a reason other than what you think. Often it is not until much later that the purpose is revealed, and sometimes it never is. It is not always necessary to understand why something happens, but it is necessary to determine what YOU are going to do about it.

- Practice kindness and accept it from others.

- Express gratitude toward others as well as yourself. Focus on the things you have, not on what you don't have. Celebrate your successes rather than diminishing them.

- The transfer of energy is real. Plant yourself in healthy, positive environments. If you are inviting negativity in, rethink that choice. If the negative environment is in your head, work hard to rewrite the script.

- Face your fear—avoiding it doesn't make it go away.

- We are aware of only a fraction of our thoughts. The subconscious mind is quite active, and if you feel it is trying to come to the surface, be open to exploring how to help it along.

- Growth is messy and ugly and painful, but the result is often something beautiful.

- Your mind matters and you are in control of it. Be a Better Being and steer it in the positive direction.

Chapter Seven

BALANCE YOUR ACT

ONE OF THE MOST POPULAR trainings I teach is on the topic of work-life balance. I find it so interesting that "work" and "life" are viewed as two separate things. If you are in your income-earning years (and not the recipient of a large trust fund), work is PART of your life. Of course, it is going to take up a large chunk of your day, but unfortunately what has happened is we now accept this idea that we work all the time—it has become normalized. There are more demands, more expectations, and more opportunities than ever before, and yet we still only have 24 hours in the day. How can we possibly find the time for all the things we need to do, plus all the things we want to do, AND still end up a healthy human being? The reality is, you probably can't.

Yes, I said it—you can't have it ALL.

I wish I could:

eat whatever I want

rarely exercise

buy anything I want whenever I want it

go out to every social event that looks fun and interesting

be informed on every aspect of my friends'
lives and happenings in the world

work a high-paying job that requires little time and effort

do everything to please everyone

AND . . . still be a happy, healthy, productive, high functioning being!

This, my friends, is not reality.

So, what's a girl (or guy) to do? How do we structure our days/weeks/lives to find time for the necessities of life while also finding joy, purpose, and fulfillment? You have already started, because you are reading this book! What comes next is identifying your GOALS, VALUES, and PRIORITIES. If you are spending time, money, and energy on things that don't really matter, or on things that do not align with your values, or in ways that are not getting you closer to your goals, you are wasting those resources. This will result in your feeling overwhelmed, unappreciated, unfulfilled, and out of balance. It will also most likely cause a deterioration in your physical, mental, and emotional well-being. Something is going to give! You will be STRESSED!

Your productivity will suffer.

Your relationships will suffer.

Your health will suffer.

To really clarify what your Priorities and Values are, fill out the following worksheet. I know some of you are thinking, "I know what my priorities are; I don't need to fill this out." YES, YOU DO! I have taught this class hundreds of times and watched people struggle with the actual words that define their priorities and values. Think of priorities as things that have an elevated level of importance and values as standards of behavior or characteristics that are held in high regard.

PRIORITIES AND VALUES WORKSHEET INSTRUCTIONS

Once you have made the lists of your priorities and values, fill in the two circles with all things that take up your time on a given day. The top circle should represent how you are currently spending your time, and the bottom circle will depict how you would like to be spending your time. Please keep the bottom circle based in reality. If it is not realistic to spend 24 hours of your day sitting on a beach, resist the temptation to live in that fantasy. If that IS in the realm of possibility, draw it— then let's figure out how to make it happen!

Most people find it helpful to divide the circle into a pie chart but feel free to create whatever makes sense to you. I also encourage you to invite people you share time and space with to fill out their own worksheets. This will provide valuable insight into the dynamics of certain relationships and may foster a more supportive and nurturing environment.

PRIORITIES

1. _____
2. _____
3. _____
4. _____
5. _____
6. _____
7. _____
8. _____
9. _____
10. _____

HOW ARE YOU SPENDING YOUR TIME?

VALUES

1. _____
2. _____
3. _____
4. _____
5. _____
6. _____
7. _____
8. _____
9. _____
10. _____

HOW WOULD YOU LIKE TO SPEND YOUR TIME?

An important step in creating balance is to assess your current status. The Satisfaction Survey is designed to do just that. There are many layers to this worksheet, and the step-by-step instructions will guide you through the process. At the end you will have all the tools to create an action plan for elevating your level of satisfaction.

SATISFACTION SURVEY

For each statement determine whether you:

Strongly agree	5
Agree	4
Neutral	3
Disagree	2
Strongly Disagree	1

Physical health is important to me _____

I am satisfied with the state of my health _____

My attitude impacts my outcome _____

I find the positive in every situation _____

I need external praise to feel successful _____

I feel supported in my pursuits _____

I prefer to be the decision maker _____

I am making most of the decisions in my life _____

I need to be heard and validated _____

I have a safe environment to express ideas _____

Financial stability is a must _____

I am comfortable with my financial situation _____

I need time to do my own thing _____

I take time to renew my spirit _____

I value solid
friendships _____

Making contributions fuels my
motivation _____

Defined purpose enables
me to thrive _____

I perform better when
I feel good _____

I prefer to be in a
nurturing relationship _____

I function well when
I am at peace _____

I get bored if I am
not challenged _____

I need everything
to be perfect _____

I easily adapt
to change _____

I utilize stress management
tools effectively _____

I measure success by
material assets _____

I have enough high-quality
friendships _____

I feel like a valuable member at home _____
I feel like a valuable member at work _____

I recognize
my purpose _____

I take time for
self-care _____

I have a positive
partner in my life _____

I am able to let go of what
I cannot control _____

I have avenues
toward growth _____

I do the best I can with
what I've got _____

I have resources to
reach out to for help _____

I am always
stressed out _____

I am pleased with the
pace of my results _____

SATISFACTION SURVEY INSTRUCTIONS

1. Once you have assigned each line value, determine your satisfaction. If you agree with a statement in the first column, and the rank of that statement in the second column is lower, that would indicate an area for improvement.

   For example:
   My Health is important to me 5
   I am satisfied with my health 3
   In this case you may want to create an action plan to modify behaviors that are necessary to elevate your level of satisfaction with your physical health.

   I easily adapt to change **2**
   I have resources available and reach out for help **4**
   In this case, you have recognized a challenge and have tools in place to help you with this. There is no sense of urgency for change in this area.

2. Circle any statements where you are less than satisfied with your current status. Next, put a star by those that you are in control of changing. Do not worry about how difficult it may be, but rather if YOU HAD to do something about it, you could.

3. Next, look at all the items you starred. Most likely you have starred all circled statements. Yes, you are in control of all of these things! You are not necessarily in control of the outcome, but you CAN do something about every item on the list. Put a GIANT SMILEY

FACE next to any items you are READY and WILL-
ING to do something about.

4. Let's first address those items that are starred, but
    have no smiley face. What are you going to do with
    things you know you can change, but are not ready
    or willing right now? Often these are the things we
    obsess about, beat ourselves up about and cause us to
    feel deflated and defeated. It's OK if you can't tackle
    it right now. It's OK if you decide that the work you
    need to put into it is just not worth the time, mon-
    ey or energy, for the possibility of the outcome you
    say you want. But if this is the case, you need to do
    something with it. If you allow it to continue to clog
    your mind and drain your energy, possibly use up
    your money, you won't have the capacity to do the
    things you ARE ready for. We will revisit this a bit
    later, so you have strategies to free up the space and
    energy that will allow you to make real progress.

5. Now, let's get back to business! Those areas with a
    smiley face are waiting for you to take action! You
    are READY and WILLING to change behaviors to
    elevate your level of satisfaction so it matches how
    important you say this is. If something got a high
    rank in column 1, it should also appear on your list of
    Priorities and Values. Double check---if it's not there,
    this is a good time to add it to the list. Pick one or
    two and write a SMART goal to outline exactly how
    you plan to facilitate change.

Are you ready to stop trying and start doing? These steps will get you on your way. Small changes lead to big results, but you have to START. Do not go one more day, week, or year without making a change. Once you pass on the opportunity to make a better choice, you don't get that opportunity back. Slow progress IS progress, and as long as you are moving in the right direction, that is success. You will discover this, but I'll let you in on a little secret: If you make a change in one area, it will have a domino effect in several other areas. That is what is SO beautiful about the whole process. One choice affects us on multiple levels, so although it might look like you have a lot to do, changing one little thing might actually take care of many others. Trust me, it really does work this way! This is the method of a Better Being.

I want to circle back for a moment to address those things that are hanging over or cluttering up your head. If you are not satisfied with something, the options are:

A. Complain about it   B. Change it   C. Leave it.

Complaining is easy but not healthy, and it gets you nowhere. Change would be healthy, but it is hard, and you have already determined that you are not willing to change this, at least not right now. Leaving it is also hard . . . but the only option left for a Better Being.

In Chapter Six we spent a great deal of time working on re-writing the script and changing the narrative. In many instances the best choice is to leave it, to accept what is, or reassess the degree of importance the issue has on your level of overall satis-faction. Let it go! You may need to reframe and gain perspective in order to bring it into balance. The specific words you use can either be empowering or they can leave you feeling like a vic-tim. Remember, you are making the CHOICE to take no action. Choice is power and power is valuable. If and when you deter-mine you are ready for change, you'll know what to do, but for now, take a deep breath, stand tall, and forge on with changes you are ready to make!

STRESS AND YOUR HEALTH

If we are not managing our stressors in a healthy way, we end up in a state of chronic response. Hormones remain out of balance because they have not had the opportunity to reset. When we are in a state of hormonal imbalance, any and all systems will be affected. Every physical and mental health issue a human being faces is either rooted in or made worse by chronic stress. Those responses that happen in an acute phase of stress, those that allow us to survive, are now leading us down the road to illness.

The Stress Response

In order to survive the threat or take on excess demand, our bodies must adapt to the new situation. Physical changes are triggered by the fight-or-flight response. These changes occur on a hormonal level and set in motion a flurry of activity to allow the body to perform in a way it cannot perform under normal circumstances. The primary hormones involved are adrenaline and cortisol. When the brain perceives a threat of any kind (something dangerous that could cause me to die), the adrenal glands kick out adrenaline and cortisol. This serves a critical purpose when faced with a real danger. Back in the day big beasts wanted to eat us, so it was necessary to have intense focus, decreased self-awareness, and increased blood pressure and blood sugar. In preparation for a fight, we tighten our chests, raise our shoulders, and brace our necks. We have many ways to survive various threats, but these are supposed to be temporary conditions. We fight or flee, we survive, and we move on. Our lifestyles used to have built-in recovery mechanisms. We ate real food that provided powerful medicine to heal the body; we didn't eat fake food that causes our immune system to constantly flush out toxins; we hunted and gathered all day long, which was very hard physical work. All this great work took place during the daylight, and when darkness fell, we hid for protection to avoid danger. During the darkness, the brain was allowed to release brain chemicals like melatonin and adenosine, which made us drowsy. We had plenty of opportunity for rest, repair, recovery, and hormonal reset while we slept. Then, the sun came up, which triggered a release of adrenaline and cortisol. Cortisol instructed glucose and triglycerides from stores in the liver to be released into the blood-stream so we had some fuel to think and function. To circulate that fuel, cortisol also instructed an increase in heart rate and blood pressure. We then went about our day, hunting, gathering, eating that real food we worked so hard for, until darkness again fell.

DOES THIS LOOK LIKE YOUR LIFE TODAY?

Cortisol

You can think of cortisol as the project manager of the fight-or-flight response. It tells other hormones what to do based on the nature of the threat. Remember, ANY threat or perceived threat will trigger the release of cortisol.

Big beasts wanting to eat us, another tribe trying to take our land, wounds and injuries, bacteria, a drought or a famine—these were all real threats to human life and triggered a release of cortisol. To be hunted by a beast was probably a scary thing! It was best to not spend too much time thinking about the situation but rather to react—and fast! Don't think, just do! To fight another human we must act big and tough—puff out the chest, grit the teeth, and raise those shoulders. During injury, cortisol triggers the release of the pro-inflammatory eicosanoids to protect us from further harm and start the healing process. Once the threat is under control, cortisol triggers the release of the anti-inflammatory eicosanoids to shut down the process. Starvation and famine were common for our ancestors. When there is a food shortage, the body begins to conserve energy so it can last as long as possible. In addition, to protect your organs, cortisol will direct fat to be stored around your midsection. Hopefully, we get back to feasting mode well before we have lost so much weight that the organs are actually in danger! All of these functions were necessary and helpful for our survival back then. Because our lives now look NOTHING like they used to, we find ourselves in a state of chronic stress, which leads to chronic hormonal imbalance, which leads to NOTHING good.

Mental and Emotional Health

Mental and emotional well-being are often negatively affected when we are stressed. Do you find yourself irritable or short-tempered? How about a lack of concentration or an inability to make decisions? Anxiety, depression, and social withdrawal are common. Reactions to situations are typically negative—born out of fear or the feeling we need to defend ourselves. When cortisol is released, it can shut down the thought processes of the brain, which when faced with a beast about to eat you was quite helpful. In most situations today, reacting rather than thinking then responding usually leads to more negativity and stress.

Brain Function

Some people find it difficult to concentrate and have a hard time completing tasks. The memory seems to go by the wayside under stress, and you find yourself easily confused. This is most likely occurring because chronically elevated cortisol destroys synapses. These are the bridges that connect neurons in the brain, which is how thoughts are transmitted.

Metabolism

Although metabolism is boosted during fight or flight, it plummets under chronic stress. Not knowing how long it will be forced to continue to fight, your body begins to conserve energy. This means you are not burning calories as you should, which can lead to weight gain. In addition, if you are not using the fuel provided, you may end up with high blood sugar, leading to diabetes or high triglycerides and increasing your risk for heart disease.

Immune Response

It is extremely taxing on the immune system to be constantly fighting. While overcoming a true injury—a cut, a broken arm, a virus—cortisol has an anti-inflammatory effect. Once the injury is healed sufficiently to no longer pose a threat to life, cortisol completes the loop by shutting off the release of inflammatory hormones. If the body is under continual attack, inflammation is now chronic. Think of all the ways we injure ourselves today. Yes, we still deal with wounds and bacteria, but anything the body perceives as an injury or as potentially harmful will cause inflammation. High blood pressure is an injury to the arteries causing extra stress with each heartbeat. Some types of cholesterol, the very small particles that can burrow in between the lining of your artery walls, cause injury. Chronic high blood sugar levels, or even consuming too much sugar at one time, can be damaging to your arteries. Those glucose molecules are very rough and jagged, and when they flood the bloodstream, they rub the artery wall, similar to rubbing sandpaper on the back of your hand. If we consume substances the body doesn't recognize (fake fat, artificial sweeteners, chemicals, pesticides, etc.), it will try to protect you from them. All of this, and much more, leads us to a state of chronic inflammation. When the immune system is constantly working to protect and defend, it can't always perform its basic functions. Frequent illness, infections, rashes, joint pain, and autoimmune flare-ups are just a few of the consequences of unmanaged stress.

Physical Systems

A physical response to a stressor is quite normal. It is ingrained in us to posture for the fight or brace for the pain. This leads to tense muscles, headaches, and nervous tics. As cortisol destroys the lining of your digestive tract and stomach wall, many people experience digestive and intestinal disorders as well.

Sleep Disturbance

There are many reasons why we can't sleep, and stress usually tops the list! Yes, the busy mind keeps us awake, but cortisol is also playing a role. When we wake up in the morning, adrenaline and cortisol are released to help get us going. Cortisol level is supposed to gradually decrease throughout the day so it is at the lowest when you go to sleep. When our triggers send us into fight or flight, cortisol is released. Cortisol stimulates us into action— difficult to sleep when you have a hormone coursing through your body to keep you alert. In addition, if you have ignored the message of adenosine, that brain chemical that makes you sleepy, the brain thinks you MUST NEED to stay awake. You must be the night watch whose job it is to tell the tribe that danger is approaching. Or you are actually fighting or fleeing danger. Back in the day these were the only reasons you were awake in the darkness, but today cortisol will still be released to aid in your survival.

Adrenal Fatigue and Failure

Waiting for the threat to go away is a lot to ask of the human body. We weren't designed to stay in a heightened state of response for an extended period of time. Eventually something is going to give. Your body will do whatever it can to survive, but eventually the adrenal glands start wearing out. It begins with adrenal fatigue, with low levels of adrenaline and cortisol being produced. You will be tired and lethargic. Eventually the adrenal glands are done, so the thyroid takes over to try to keep you going. If we ignore the body's warning signs and continue in a state of unchecked chronic stress, the thyroid gets out of balance. This sets in motion another level of chaos for the body and a very long road back to optimal health and wellness.

MANAGING STRESS

Hopefully, by now you fully appreciate how significantly unmanaged stress can affect your physical and mental health. Are you ready to get a handle on it? To stress less? Let's keep it simple for now. Your goal at the very basic level is to not allow a release of cortisol if it is not necessary. For most of us, true fight-or-flight situations are extremely rare. Our stressors are really NOT actual threats to our lives, but that's what our brains think because we are programmed for survival. Your job is to retrain your brain and minimize other behaviors the body could perceive as a threat.

First you must identify your specific triggers. In what situations do you find yourself getting angry, annoyed, or frustrated, or having negative thoughts or feelings? Each of these reactions means cortisol is being released, so you'll want to find a different way to respond to a trigger. I think at the very least, training yourself to breathe can prevent the immediate (and probably negative) reaction. Breathing will also minimize the cortisol release and get oxygen to your brain—helpful for thinking! The concepts in the "Mind Matters" chapter (Chapter Six) are all helpful for rewiring your brain; refer to it if you need some reminders.

We often invite our stressors in. monitoring the news or social media, getting involved in someone else's drama, and voluntarily being around negative people are sources of stress you are choosing to introduce into your environment. These can all be time and energy suckers, so rethinking their value and importance may free up time and energy for other things.

In addition to preventing the release of cortisol, we need to regularly engage in behaviors that will help repair and reset our bodies from the fight-or-flight response. It will come as no shock that these behaviors lead to "the healthy lifestyle."

- eat healthy food more often than not—PFF every 2–4 hours, most calories early and often, and fewer calories as you get closer to bedtime

- move your body as much as you can, as hard as you can, as often as you can

- establish a routine for quality sleep

- participate only in positive environments—home, work, friends, and in your head

I know this chapter covered a tremendous amount of information, but I can't STRESS enough how important it is to recognize the dangers of chronic stress. Overriding your ingrained response, training your brain to do something that isn't natural, is very difficult. But it IS possible. The stress response sets us up for so many other challenges, from the actual physical and mental health difficulties to choices we make to cope with our stress, which usually are not healthy either! If you can prevent the fight-or-flight response from kicking in when it's not needed, so many other things will fall into place. I hope this chapter, together with the previous one, helped you realize just how much power you actually have. You are ready to harness that power by making intentional choices that work to your advantage rather than letting everything spiral down a path where you feel you have no control.

Consider the following homework to keep you moving in the right direction:

1. Work with your triggers:

    • specifically identify your triggers—give them real names (people, places, things)

    • write down what your natural response is to each trigger

    • if you recognize that it is fight or flight—anger, irritation, frustration, negativity—come up with an alternative response that will prevent the release of cortisol

2. Complete the worksheets

3. Create your SMART goals

FINAL THOUGHTS

You are in control of you—what you think and feel and say and do. You cannot control what anyone else thinks or feels or says or does. You cannot control what comes your way, but you do get to decide what you are going to do with it. You are not in control of outcomes, only behaviors. Breathe, walk away, redirect the conversation, or set a boundary. Learn to say no. If something or someone is not serving you in a healthy, productive way, eliminate it or remove yourself from the environment. These changes are hard, but I am willing to bet the way things are going for you now is hard too. Pick your hard. Be a Better Being.

Chapter Eight

ARE YOU FEEDING YOUR FEELINGS?

HUMANS EXPERIENCE SO MANY emotions—happy, sad, bored, angry, excited—and it seems every one of them is better when experienced with food. I don't know about you, but when I am reaching for food to enhance, subdue, or avoid a feeling, I'm not reaching for chicken and broccoli. I know, weird, right? My go-to would be some combined form of fat and sugar—I LOVE SWEETS! I love chips and fries and pizza and pasta, and enjoy some versions of adult beverages too, but I LOVE SWEETS. I used to say I was addicted to sugar, that I "craved" it, but then I got real with myself. I am not addicted to sugar; I just REALLY love it.

How, why, and when did this love of sweets start? I am going to blame my sweet tooth on my grandmother. She was a traditional German woman who created glorious confections. There were always homemade pies, pound cake, and several varieties of traditional German cookies out on the counter in her house. A sweet after every meal and during break time was standard practice. I did not grow up in her house or anywhere near her house. In fact, I only saw my grandparents for a few weeks each year, but she passed this norm on to my father. We always had cookies, pie, and delicious treats in the house, some store-bought and others made over the weekend with my mom and sister. Dinner was not complete until dad had a "cookie to wash down the last bit of milk." There was nothing better than coming in from a cold winter day, the hard work over of stacking firewood or playing mechanic assistant to my dad, and being treated to hot chocolate and something sweet. In addition, my mom is Dutch. Do you know anything about Dutch chocolate? Well, let me tell you, it is heavenly. The discovery of Vander Veen's, a Dutch store in Michigan, meant we could have all the amazing treats of my mother's childhood delivered to our door in a matter of days. We had a "chocolate cabinet." No joke—this was the cabinet in the kitchen that literally housed nothing but deliciousness. I swear it had a magnetic pull on me! On weekends I always looked forward to afternoon tea. This is a tradition in Europe that got lost across the pond but one that held strong in my family. Of course, afternoon tea meant an assortment of chocolates and cookies, because clearly you can't drink tea without something sweet to accompany it! It was a special tradition. One that I know few other people in my world got to experience because in my small Wisconsin town, nobody else had a foreign mom. It was also fun because it meant I got to eat chocolate in the middle of the day.

None of this would really be an issue if I had been a normal kid. And here is where I think a lot of my future issues with food began. I wasn't normal. By sixth grade I was heavily involved in gymnastics, practicing six days a week for three to four hours a day. As for many girls my age, the growing body can be difficult to deal with, and when a growing body does not exactly help you excel in the sport you love, the difficulties compound. The desire to participate in life in the same ways my friends did—which often involved being around a lot of fun food—conflicted with the need to stay thin. This led to my either avoiding social activities or building up anxiety when I was in the situations. I was often so focused on the food that was around that I "shouldn't" be having, that it was ALL I wanted. Sometimes I was "strong" and said no in that moment, only to go home and raid the chocolate cabinet. Other times I gave in then spent the next day or two hating myself for doing so. I would go for a few days barely eating anything to compensate for the hole I dug, which led to eventually overeating for a few days. And so began the ugly cycle. Along the way, various questions, suggestions, instructions, and demands were intersecting in my brain, and the result was chaos. On any given day I might have heard the following:

> *"Why aren't you eating? You're so skinny; you need to eat."*

> *"What did you eat today? Should you really be eating that?"*

> *"Girls, it's time for weigh-in. Get your weight down by the next time you come to practice."*

> *"See those girls over there? They were once small like you. That's going to be you soon if you don't do something about it."*

> *"Do you want to go get a 'sin'?" (This will become clear below.)*

I do not blame anyone for my subsequent issues with food. I know people had good intentions and were trying to support me in the ways they knew how. They wanted me to be the best gymnast I could be, and the threat of weight gain was not only going to limit my abilities, but it posed a safety issue as well. There were plenty of girls on my team who got the same messages and did not get a jacked-up relationship with food. This is one of the complexities people face—whether you are trying to support a child with athletic aspirations or just trying to raise healthy human beings. Each person processes and internalizes information differently. What ends up shaping our own relationship with food is multifaceted, not solely a product of environment but also of personality. In addition I think we now know a lot more about how to properly fuel the body, whether it is for weight loss or optimal performance. If I had known PFF could have been my BFF, and how not eating was just setting me up for failure, I may not have struggled for so many years.

Talking about food is a sensitive subject for many people and continued to be for me well after I ended gymnastics. As I mentioned previously, after I quit, I got FAT. You can probably guess how I accomplished that—eating whatever I wanted, whenever I wanted. The day I quit, I put a note on my coach's car window telling her I was not coming back to the gym. I then went to the nearest Dairy Queen and ordered the largest Blizzard they made—peanut butter crunch with extra peanut butter. Yes, this is "the sin." I ate that on my way to another DQ and ordered the same thing. Just for good measure I hit up the third DQ and had one more! Yup, it's true. Yucky and embarrassing to admit but true. It was so delicious and incredibly freeing! I didn't have to get into a leotard or on the scale for anyone, and it was no longer anyone's business to question what I was or was not eating. It was a giant middle finger to the world and anyone in it who had anything to say about my weight. To say I didn't care what the outcome was going to be is probably not accurate. I think it was more like I was in denial of what the outcome was going to be. I imagined I would just go about this way for a while to get it out of my system, then I'd get on a "sensible" diet. Of course, that's not the way it goes—ever! Not surprisingly, weight was coming on quite rapidly, then the dread and self-loathing kicked in. By now, it was clear to everyone I was gaining weight, and so the commentary began. Some of the comments were out of concern, some were pure judgment, but I was having none of it. At this point, I didn't care.

OK, I cared. I just didn't really know what to do about it. I exercised more, but you can't exercise your way out of all the horrible choices I was making. I dieted—and we all know how well that works! I avoided situations where I would be tempted to indulge, but that becomes very isolating and lonely. To say it was a difficult time in my life is an understatement. Around this time I was getting ready to move to Hawaii for college, and I thought this would be the fresh start I needed. HA! A fresh start means not knowing anyone and to socialize means to be around food. ALL. THE. TIME. Food is part of culture and a way to express love. The aloha spirit embraces all of this, and the joy and happiness I felt by being included was wonderful. You can't be rude and not participate, and being an outsider already, I didn't want to stand out even more! I had many groups of friends—from locals who truly made me part of their ohana (family) and the residents at the off-campus dorm (many who were also new to the island) to the mix of locals, transplants, and transients I worked with at my various jobs. In every case food was central to our shared experience. Add to that being in college—going out and all that comes with it. Eating, drinking, staying out too late, going out for brunch—basically doing what most college kids do. Obviously, this was a disastrous environment for anyone trying to lose weight!

Fast-forward to when I went home for my friend's wedding, the real turning point for my weight-loss journey. As the weight came off from all my daily walking and minimal exposure to excess amounts of food, I knew this was my chance to make some real changes. The concepts of these changes are outlined in Steps 1–8 in Chapter Two, so I am going to focus on the solutions for your individual challenges when it comes to your relationship with food.

FOOD AND YOUR MOOD

Label your emotion. Use WAITE (Why am I tempted to eat?); if the answer is bored, sad, lonely, anxious, stressed, etc., sit with the feeling for 5 minutes and contemplate how food is going to affect this emotion. Are you trying to avoid the feeling, comfort yourself, or perhaps literally change the way you feel by creating an altered state of mind? We know this is a temporary fix and often leads to feeling much worse later on. It is easy to mask a feeling with food or alcohol, but the feeling is still there. It makes sense that if you feed your feelings, they grow—and yet we are most likely trying to accomplish the exact opposite! Try these strategies:

Bored

Create a list of things you need to do or enjoy doing and implement one as a substitute for searching the fridge. Are you truly bored or is it actually procrastination? I used to think I ate out of boredom but then realized food was a more interesting or entertaining option than whatever it was I needed to do (study, clean, work on a project). I've learned to stave off procrastination by chunking "to dos" into small blocks of manageable time. Perhaps I will clean one little area or commit to a task for 15 minutes, with a clear start and stop time. More often than not, I do more than originally planned, and I avoid eating when it isn't necessary! Maybe a quick walk in fresh air is all you need to get over the moment. Until these replacements are firmly ingrained in your brain, I encourage you to have the list handy as a reminder of what you are going to do instead of eat.

Sad/Lonely

For many people, food can be a comforting friend—it is there any time you want it and never lets you down. Obviously it is not a healthy substitute for human interaction, so get out there and socialize! I know what you are thinking—socializing often involves food, but it doesn't have to. Suggest a walk with a friend or a shopping outing. Maybe it can involve food, and you find a healthy restaurant or cook a meal together. This is a really tough one because if you are sad or lonely you may not feel like putting on a happy face, but you HAVE to. Social isolation is terrible for so many reasons, so buck up, Buttercup, and get out there!

Anxious

Anxiety can creep in for a variety of reasons and often is a response to a stress trigger. The first step is to minimize that release of cortisol by taking deep breaths and redirecting your thoughts. Hopefully, you have done the homework from the previous chapters and have been practicing these skills. I recognized I was anxious when I was waiting for something, whether it was a person to show up, a webinar I was about to teach, or a plane to arrive. Typically, there was not enough time to really do anything, so naturally food was a great filler! Now I may step out on my balcony and enjoy the view or find a cat and wake her up for no good reason or have that magazine handy that I never have time to read. Anything that does not get me too absorbed so I lose track of time is a great substitute, and I know you can find a few of your own that are suitable!

Stressed

The stress response puts you in a sugar cycle by releasing glucose into the bloodstream. It's like you've eaten a doughnut without the benefit of its deliciousness! If you have no fat or protein going into the bloodstream along with this glucose, your blood sugar will crash. This is why you reach for some version of a white, refined, processed carbohydrate or a sugary food or beverage and not steamed vegetables! Two main things are necessary to get out of "stress eating": 1) prevent the release of cortisol in the first place and 2) keep blood sugar steady throughout the day. Remember, hunger itself is a stressor, so PFF every 2–4 hours, with most of your calories early in the day, will ensure that even if you allow a stress trigger to send you into fight or flight, at least you will have protein and fat in the bloodstream when the glucose gets released—avoiding the crash! You also will want to establish the "insteads" because seeking out a treat is a habit when you feel stressed. Remove yourself from the environment, go for a walk, brew some herbal tea, perform breathing exercises, or even reach for the healthy snack you've packed. Eventually these new options will become the habit, breaking the cycle of stress eating.

YOUR RELATIONSHIP WITH FOOD

I talked a little bit about your relationship with food in Chapter Three—how we often use it as reward or punishment. "I deserve it" has a similar feeling—I deserve dessert because I ate a salad, or I deserve this meal because I've "been good" all week. There is nothing wrong with eating delicious food that isn't necessarily healthy for us, but I do think the dialogue we use surrounding those foods impacts us much more than in just that moment. Why do you think I went to Dairy Queen for a specific type of treat to start my new life without gymnastics? For so long I had sacrificed, not getting to have whatever I wanted, whenever I wanted it. I deserved this! That Blizzard was, after all, a "sin." This was how it was labeled by my coaches. Sometimes my mom would pick me up from gymnastics and say very quietly (even though we were the only ones in the car), "Do you want to go get a sin?" OF COURSE I did! Not only did I think a peanut butter crunch Blizzard with extra peanut butter was incredibly tasty, but it was forbidden and sneaky. It was fun to partake in this little bit of naughtiness with my mom. These feelings would feed certain moods. If I was feeling rebellious or like I really had worked hard or given something up, I deserved to eat whatever I wanted. There is also a bit of joy that comes from sharing a secret with someone you've participated in a crime with! OK, seriously, eating ice cream is not a crime, nor is it a sin. It's actually just an enjoyable part of life for a lot of people. Although I felt I deserved to eat these things, I sure was not pleased with the outcome it led to, and I would almost immediately feel terrible about my choice. The long-term effect of the weight gain was equally as damaging, and the only remedy was to change my perception of food. Food is just food! I can have anything I want, but I have to balance that with the outcome I want. It has caused me to become a picky eater, making sure that if something is not going to help me achieve my outcome, it is totally NOT worth it! You need to decide in those moments what is more important—the immediate pleasure I am going to experience or the long-term goal I am striving for? It is hard to say no to things we enjoy, but it is also hard to be constantly disappointed in ourselves and not live the life we say we want. Pick your hard.

Food Is Love

We have probably all experienced the scenario where someone went to great lengths to create a meal or our favorite dessert, or simply surprises us with a treat. Because someone was thoughtful and took time and effort, it would be rude to reject the offering. Most likely we would really enjoy eating it, which makes it even more difficult to say no! Food is often an expression of love, but it is rarely expressed with a plate of mixed greens. If we say yes at every opportunity, the result may not be so enjoyable. This is one of the situations where you might want to have a conversation to help get over this hurdle. How to handle a saboteur is discussed in Chapter Two, so take some time to think about what this discussion will sound like. I think it is best to come at it from a place of appreciation. Acknowledge that you appreciate their kindness, but you would appreciate it even more if they stopped offering. If they are genuinely trying to express love, your request will be honored. If it is a situation you are not comfortable confronting, you will have to come up with alternative solutions. You might accept the offering and at first chance get rid of it. Oh no—we can't waste food! Yes, we can. Really. It'll be OK. You may already be wasting food, because food that you eat and don't truly need is also wasteful. It can go in the garbage or it can turn into garbage—your call.

Ultimately you are responsible for your choices, so if you are accepting the offer so as not to hurt another person's feelings or to draw attention, YOU are making that choice. What you put in your mouth has zero effect on the other person's goals, but it has a major effect on yours.

If you are the food pusher, please stop! When your offer has been declined, accept that and move on. If you are a pusher who won't stop, my guess is you are intentionally sabotaging someone's efforts to overcome this challenge. It really is not kind, and I hope at some point you have your own breakthrough to discover why you do this. This may lead you on your own journey to be a Better Being.

It's Not Fair

"It's not fair that my husband can eat whatever he wants and not gain weight." "It's not fair that my friends can eat whatever they want and still look great." "It's not fair that all these skinny bitches have no problems with food issues." I hear these things all the time and I've already addressed how I thought it wasn't fair, but I also think, quite often, assumptions are being made that are totally off base. It's possible those skinny bitches DO have problems with food. Maybe your friend eats whatever she wants and looks great but is a mess in the head. Just because your husband doesn't gain weight doesn't mean the food he's eating is not going to lead to other health issues down the road. What someone else is or is not doing has zero relevance to you, so stop comparing. Life's not fair. Get over it.

I'll Worry About It Later

"This one cookie, one meal, one day of eating garbage, won't matter—I'll worry about it later!" The thing is, this statement is true! One item, one meal, or one day most likely is not going to have a huge impact on the long-term result, but this self-talk usually does not happen only occasionally. Your strategy here is to remember that later comes a lot more quickly than you think, and by the time you get around to it, there may be A LOT to worry about. Decide if it's worth it, and if it isn't, pass!

If it is worth it, enjoy, but don't allow one choice or one meal or one day to drag on and on and on. Set some boundaries around your pleasure foods. I have a 72-hour rule for these situations. I can have something every 72 hours, and it may be a choice, a meal, or a whole day of fun food, but I will not have another choice, meal, or day like that for at least 72 hours. It has allowed me to go into situations with a clear mindset of what the plan is. There are endless opportunities to partake, and I used to go in saying, "I'm going to try to be good." Guess what—it rarely, if ever, worked out, because trying is not a strategy! I generally know what kinds of events are going on and what the food situation will look like, and I determine which of those occasions I am going to stay clean and which I am going to eat whatever I want. This is helpful for getting over all-or-nothing thinking, which often leads to self-sabotage.

TRIGGERS

Particular situations can trigger us to eat a certain way. Identifying these triggers will be critical for long-term success, because most likely these will be part of your life for a good long time.

People

Do you eat a certain way around some people and a different way around others? At many points in my life I was around two distinct types—those who were leading a lifestyle similar to mine where food is fun and more is better, and those who were leading the fairly healthy lifestyle that I envied. Early on in my commitment to making serious changes in my habits, I knew I was going to have to limit how often I hung out with my fun food friends. The summer I went home for my friend's wedding was a catalyst in this process, and I knew I wanted to carry this momentum with me back to school. I decided since I was already walking twelve to fifteen miles, I might as well sign up for the Honolulu Marathon, which is held in early December. I would need to get up early to train, so this was a perfect excuse to say no to going out at night. Weekends were the time for the long runs so that eliminated the option of going out for breakfast as well. This strategy was great for me because it squashed the peer pressure that often comes when you say no to something you had previously participated in. It also paved the way for easier handling of future situations. I did not continue to say no forever, but by the time the marathon was over, I had set a new expectation, so it didn't seem odd if I declined an invitation.

I have a bit of a unique challenge because of my profession. I am the "healthy" one in most of my circles and frequently find myself responding to someone's comment about what I may or may not be eating at the time. It has always been interesting to me that people think I care or will judge what they are eating ("Michelle, don't look at my plate") or when someone is astonished that I have seconds on dessert and feels the need to announce it.

Equally puzzling is when I am eating "healthy" food and it must be pointed out—"oh you are so good to order a salad." I know when you are trying to make healthier choices you will get some of this same reaction. I used to get really irritated about these interactions but have learned that it is them, not me, who has chosen to focus on food. Depending on who is saying it, and how often I've heard it from the same person, I may ignore the comment or say something a bit snarky. In recent years I have taken the opportunity to enlighten people about how their words and comments regarding what someone else is eating can make that person uncomfortable. In my experience, most people do not enjoy having someone else put the spotlight on them. Unless you are the person who has been asked to support another by calling them out when making unhealthy choices, I think it is just best to keep the chatter to yourself.

Places and Events

Are there particular places where you find yourself making indulgent choices? A holiday party, the company picnic, camping, or going home for a visit or on vacation? Unless you plan to stay locked in your house (which I do not recommend), you will want to know how to deal with each of these situations. One rule always is do not "save" your calories for the occasion! All you are doing throughout the day is plunging your metabolism, kicking out cortisol, and setting yourself up for overdoing it later. Here are some ideas that have helped me stay mindful when out of my regular environment:

Survey the estate. Before you start loading your plate, have a good look at the options and make some thoughtful decisions on what you think will be worth it; don't bother with the rest. A little bit of everything turns into a LOT of food, so consider limiting choices to one or two items from each category.

Commit to eating the real foods first—protein, vegetables, cheese. When you fill up on healthy food, there is not much room for the other.

Set a start and a stop time for consumption. This is helpful for both the food and beverage intake. You don't need to eat the minute food is in front of you. If the temptation is too great, turn around and stop looking at it!

Drink lots of water! Simple and logical.

Your strategies are going to be determined by the frequency of these occasions. For many people life is a nonstop party; for others it is a rare occurrence. The main point is to determine the plan before you go. If you rely on "trying to be good" as your plan, it is not likely to work out well!

Learned Behavior

Raise your hand if you were a member of the Clean Your Plate Club. For many of our parents and grandparents the idea of wasting food was unheard of. Although it was probably necessary to encourage us as children to eat our food, this need to eat everything in front of us becomes ingrained. It wouldn't be a problem if portions were the same size as when we were kids, but we all know how the size of a dinner plate has grown, not to mention restaurant servings. You may consider using smaller dishes (other than your salad bowls!) or measuring out your food to see what a serving looks like. When at a restaurant, just know even half the meal is probably more than you need at any given time. If you seldom eat out, it is probably not an issue, but the weekly date night meal could have more than double the calories you need for an entire day! That is a deep hole to climb out of every Monday, so be thoughtful about what is worth it and what is not. Do you really need bread just because there is a basket of it on the table?

Thinking of food as reward is also a learned behavior, so you'll want to come up with other ways of rewarding yourself and the kids. Keep in mind you are shaping their relationship with food and you likely do not want them to struggle with issues they way you have.

Habits and Associations

When was the last time you saw a movie in the theater without eating a snack? Friday night food? Whatever it is, the food that goes along with any activity is probably not helping you get closer to your goals. Do you think you could enjoy the movie without putting food in your mouth? Give it a try. And guess what, healthy food can be fun on road trips and at tailgates too. Seriously, you should try my bean dip! You definitely should have your fun food, but maybe not only on Friday night and not every Friday night. Mix it up so this is not solidified as an expectation.

PAD YOUR ENVIRONMENT FOR SUCCESS

The only way to truly overcome emotional eating is to enhance your skills as the gatekeeper. If you eat what is around you, don't put food around you that you are trying not to eat. I know this is obvious, and yet so often people tell me stories about how they gave in to the chips and cookies and ice cream. My first question is always, "Why is it in the house?" Do not be your own saboteur! Make the Four Ps your way of life to make sure you always have a healthy option in front of you—one you like. When it is an environment you do not control (work, a social gathering, a cruise, being with a saboteur), it is the environment in your HEAD that may need work. Who is your support? How are you going to deal with the situation? What's your WHY?

This chapter may not resonate with everyone, and if you are someone who does not use food as therapy, a lot of what is written might not make sense. Trust me when I say, you are the exception! I hope there was still some useful information that helps you understand someone else's challenge surrounding food issues. If you were nodding along at every sentence, welcome to my tribe! I am happy to tell you it is possible to break the psychological addiction to food. If you are ready to no longer allow your mood to choose your food, here are some things to consider:

1. Define your relationship with food.

2. Identify particular triggers and create a strategy for each one.

3. Practice WAITE (Why am I tempted to eat?)

4. Rewrite your internal dialogue surrounding food choices.

FINAL THOUGHTS

If the ONLY things you enjoyed were also the things that helped you prevent disease and reach your goals, there would have been no need for this chapter. This has already been addressed a few times, but it is SO critical for success that it bears repeating. Because we tend to make the poor choice in the moment then spend a lot of time regretting it, it is best to prevent that impulsive choice! In that moment, you have to stop and ask yourself if it's worth it. If it is not, move on. If it is, eat it, savor it, and love it, but recognize it can't always be "worth it" and still have the outcome you desire. If you are reaching for food in response to an emotion, ask yourself the following questions:

What feeling am I trying to avoid?

What feeling will I have after?

What can I do instead that will make me feel better?

If your choices relate to a certain attitude you have, define it then change your attitude. This may very well be the most difficult part of the journey for some of you because there are many layers, but you have to get to the root cause of why you are making choices that are leading you in the wrong direction. This may require getting down into some issues you'd rather not address, and if so, I encourage you to seek professional guidance. You can know everything there is to know about nutrition—what foods to eat and what to avoid to help reach your goals—but it won't create a lasting result if you are using food as therapy. Food is fun, and it is forever going to be part of your culture and your life. This chapter is not intended to have you eliminate what brings you joy; in fact, it is quite the opposite! A Better Being has the knowledge and power to balance the choices between health and pleasure, allowing you to be healthy in body, mind, and spirit.

Chapter Nine

GOOD NIGHT NOW!

HOW DID YOU SLEEP LAST NIGHT? No, really, how did you sleep? I've spent years asking this question to those around me who always seem to get a good night's sleep. What's the secret? People who have no trouble sleeping don't give it a second thought. But there are so many things that need to go right (including balancing eleven brain chemicals) to get that good night of sleep, I think it's amazing anyone does! I have come to believe sleep is like anything else—some people are naturally better at it than others. As a kid, I was the one at the slumber parties who was up, ready to go, at 6:00 a.m. Let me tell you, parents were not so thrilled. Growing up, I remember lying awake, unable to fall asleep, for what seemed like forever. I was certain I was missing out on some kind of fun. I always wondered how my sister could sleep sooooo late, even on Christmas morning. She would tell me, "Just wait until you get older and you'll be sleeping in too." Nope, never happened. By the time I moved away for college, things were getting especially interesting. Sleep talking and sleepwalking became regular occurrences. Japanese was my foreign language of choice, and my roommate would tell me I'd sit straight up in the middle of the night and start speaking Japanese (more fluently than when I was awake). I would often find my way to the stairwell at the opposite end of our dorm hall and have conversations with friends as they were coming home from a fun night out. On several occasions I woke up to find myself sleeping on the floor outside someone else's door. I had no recollection of any of these events, but it turns out I was a pretty social, conversational person while completely asleep. At the time, I thought this was funny, odd, weird. It made for great stories but was also a bit scary. I wish I had been more interested in figuring out WHY this was happening, but eventually it became less frequent then ceased altogether. I now know that change, stress, irregular sleep patterns, and chronic sleep deprivation are triggers for this type of nighttime activity.

These are just a few of the challenges I've had with sleep. For a period of time, I battled severe insomnia. It would take hours for me to fall asleep, then I would wake at one or two in the morning unable to fall back to sleep. This would happen several nights in a row and led to anxiety about going to bed. My quest for the magic answer to blissful sleep has led me to discover I am far from alone in this struggle. Although your challenges may be different, the root causes of sleep issues and the consequences of sleep deprivation are probably the same. When we are young, we can get away with a lot. I did well in school and had energy for gymnastics, work, and fun. I was a generally pleasant person, and any moodiness could be attributed to A) being a teenager or B) being hungry. As with many things, the older we get, the less resilient we become.

Unfortunately, societal norms, including schedule patterns

(school, work, activities, and dietary habits) and the overuse of technology, are making it increasingly difficult for children, teenagers, and adults to get the quality sleep necessary for optimal human functioning and performance. The side effect of not being tired the next day is just one small piece of why we need anywhere from 7–10 hours of quality sleep per night. This should be the time for internal rest, cellular repair, and hormonal reset. Parts of the brain and body get to relax, while other parts of the brain and body go to work. Chronic sleep deprivation can lead to increased risk for every single physical and mental health issue, because the critical functions designed to take place during various phases of our sleep cycle are either cut short or not happening at all. Sleep is actually a necessity not a luxury! Perhaps an understanding of the sleep cycle and what takes place during the various phases will motivate you to get your sleep habits on track.

THE SLEEP CYCLE

The length of a sleep cycle is unique to each individual, but typically lasts 70–110 minutes. To get an idea of yours, the next time you have the chance to take a nap, notice what time you drift off and what time you wake. Unless intentionally awakened, you will likely sleep one full cycle. The cycle consists of two parts: non-REM (stages 1–3) sleep, sometimes referred to as quiet sleep, and REM (rapid eye movement), referred to as active sleep. We need to get through four to six cycles per night for optimal functioning and hormonal release and reset. In *Stage 1*, as you are falling asleep, brain waves and muscle activity slows. This lasts about 5–10 minutes, during which you may feel jerky movements. Moving into *Stage 2*, eye movement stops, heart rate slows, and body temperature drops. There is further slowing of brain waves, with some intermittent fast waves. Your body and brain are literally preparing for rest. This stage lasts about 20 minutes and you can still be easily awakened.

Stage 3 is where you enter your deepest sleep and brain waves are slowest. In addition, blood pressure and body temperature drop to the lowest point, and breathing rate slows significantly. It is difficult to wake up during this stage, and you will be groggy and disoriented if you do so. This deep sleep is when the majority of cellular restoration is taking place and is critical for feeling refreshed in the morning. As much as 75 percent of your sleep is spent in non-REM stages. Once you enter the REM stage, body and brain activities resemble those of when you are awake. Heart rate and blood pressure increase, as do respiration and body temperature; there is also significant eye movement. This is the stage where your brain organizes thoughts and catalogues long-term memories. This is also the stage of dreaming, and it is thought the eye movement is related to us "watching" the subconscious mind. Although not fully understood, it is clear this stage is extremely critical for long-term brain health and functioning. Because REM stage is so active, we have a built-in protection to lock us down. The neurotransmitters, GABA and glycine, paralyze the limbs to prevent us from moving around and harming ourselves. For sleepwalkers and sleep talkers, there is a disturbance with this mechanism— either the neurotransmitters do not release or the messages are not received. It is often stress-induced and will pass, but it could also be due to an underlying issue with brainstem functioning or be a side effect of medications.

Sleep used to be looked upon as a passive activity, but we now know a tremendous amount of work is actually occurring! During each cycle, particular events are taking place. Release of gastric acid is reduced, slowing down digestion. Kidney filtration of sodium, potassium, and calcium is also reduced, which leads to sodium retention in the morning. Growth and reproductive hormones are released, as are melatonin, prolactin (after childbirth), and TSH. As we approach morning, we spend more time in our deep Stage 3 and REM stage, which are critical for repair and retention and why the quantity as well as the quality of your sleep are important.

Remember our friends gherlin and leptin—the hunger hormones? They are of particular interest when talking about lack of sleep and weight gain. Sleep deprivation, whether one night or chronic, can result in elevated gherlin and suppressed levels of leptin. It makes sense that if you are not sleeping, you must need fuel to either fight or flee the danger or to keep you alert for your night-watch duties. HA! Likely none of that is going on—you just aren't sleeping!

CONSEQUENCES OF POOR-QUALITY SLEEP

There really is no dispute about the health consequences associated with sleep deprivation. You are at increased risk for heart disease, diabetes, obesity, early-onset dementia, Alzheimer's, depression, anxiety—need I go on? In fact, the outcomes of inadequate sleep are similar to those of chronic stress, and it all goes back to hormones. If they have not had the chance to release or reset, or they are being released unnecessarily, every system they are involved with may be affected. We need hormones to help us sleep, and they get out of balance if we are not sleeping well. I told you they rule your world!

In the short term, we experience diminished reaction time, decreased motivation, and an inability to focus and concentrate. It is quite similar to being legally intoxicated. I am going to bet most of you would not show up to work drunk, but how many are going to work sleep deprived? You may also experience mood swings, sugar cravings, and energy slumps. If you are tired, you may turn to sugar or caffeine to keep you going and are not likely to exercise. The mood swings will eventually affect relationships, and lack of focus and motivation will impact productivity. It all sounds so lovely, right? If you think not, and would like a life of quality sleep, let's get to the root of the issue. WHY are you not sleeping?

WHAT'S THE PROBLEM?

There are many reasons why we are sleep deprived, and identifying your obstacles to healthy, quality sleep is the first step toward achieving it. I have come to realize that a good night's sleep starts in the morning. The behaviors we engage in throughout the day will either promote or obstruct our sleep that night. Let me outline a few of the basics.

Back in the day we operated on a natural day-night cycle of hunting and gathering during the day and, as darkness approached, getting quiet and hiding from all the dangers that lurked about. With that darkness, the pineal gland produced and released melatonin—one of our sleep-inducing hormones. Our movement throughout the day allowed the body to produce adenosine triphosphate, a byproduct of the glucose burned as fuel in the body. Adenosine is a brain chemical that also signals it is time for sleep. The sunrise triggered a release of adrenaline and cortisol, the two hormones that help get us going by releasing glucose and triglycerides into the bloodstream for fuel and circulating that fuel by increasing heart rate and blood pressure.

We ate real food (in appropriate amounts), which provided nutrients (think omega-3 fatty acids) that enabled the body to produce adequate amounts of melatonin. We did not eat fake food (think artificial flavor, colors and preservatives) the body had to work really hard to get rid of, and we were not over-consuming stimulants (think sugar and caffeine) which trigger a release of cortisol, keeping you alert.

We had the occasional big stressor (that big beast trying to eat us), and we did not have artificial light and physiologically and cognitively stimulating media devices. There was not much to do after dark, so when the sleepy signal came, we obeyed it.

For most people today, life looks nothing like that! In fact, it may be quite the opposite. The environment in which we live is not the one the human brain and body were designed for, so we need to do the best we can to simulate or create such an environment. We have been establishing this throughout the book, but let's review some key concepts.

DIET

Eat real food more often than not, consuming most calories early and often during the day and fewer as bedtime approaches. Because caffeine is a stimulant, releasing cortisol, cut off consumption at least 10 hours prior to going to bed. It can inhibit sleep in another way as well. Adenosine, the neurotransmitter that signals you are sleepy, needs to settle into its receptor to transmit the message. Caffeine molecules use these same receptors, essentially blocking adenosine from doing its job. If you have sleep issues, you may need to minimize intake to no more than 200 mg a day or eliminate it altogether. Since caffeine content can vary dramatically based on a variety of factors, it is best to consult the nutrition information of food and beverages you consume so you have a clear assessment of your intake. In addition, avoid alcohol (completely if possible) at least 4 hours prior to going to bed. Listen to your body and brain! If you find yourself snacking at night, it may be because you are ignoring the signals that it is time for bed. When you override the messages from adenosine and melatonin and force yourself to stay awake, you reach for some form of sugar. Instead of eating chips, chocolate, or ice cream—GO TO BED.

EXERCISE

Move your body as much as you can, as hard as you can, as often as you can. The body knows the difference between physical exertion and mental exertion. Lack of movement means you have a whole bunch of energy saved up and have little need for rest. We also want to produce adenosine so we have more of that messenger to tell us we are sleepy (we just have to follow its suggestion). It may be best to exercise early in the day so the activity does not prevent you from sleeping, but some people find it better in the evening. You have to experiment to see what is right for you.

STRESS

When the house gets quiet, the mind gets LOUD! It may be helpful to include as part of your sleep preparation routine a few minutes to brain-dump. If you don't get the thoughts out of your head, when exactly do you think they are going to converse with you? Use the skills detailed in previous chapters to redirect your thoughts when you find your mind wandering. Deep breathing with a centering, calming thought or a visual is quite effective for shutting off the mind; you just have to commit to constant practice. It will also be critical to manage your stressors during the day so as not to allow a release of cortisol when it isn't needed. This constant output of cortisol can definitely contribute to your inability to sleep well.

OVERLOADED SCHEDULE

So much to do and still only 24 hours to do it! This is the issue for today's human being. It is not realistic to think you can go nonstop all day, running on adrenaline and cortisol then lie down and get into deep restful sleep. The body does not work that way. This may require you to say no to some things you'd really like to do. It might mean you need to set some boundaries with yourself to use your time wisely and still have a routine that allows you to prepare for rest. Hopefully, the worksheets in Chapter Seven helped highlight for you how to modify the ways you are spending your time and energy.

INTERRUPTIONS

You may fall asleep, but then wake up and not be able to get back to sleep. If this is your issue, the first thing to identify is what is interrupting your slumber. A pet, child, significant other, full bladder, or an unexpected noise are common thieves of sleep. This might take major work or be a simple solution to prevent the disturbance. The full bladder was one of my issues back when I was doing a lot of personal training. I would drink water throughout my sessions, often until seven or eight at night, which, needless to say, got me up a few times. The easy remedy for me was to cut consumption 4–5 hours before bedtime. One time a night is still pretty typical, and once awake a whole bunch of things could prevent me from falling back to sleep. I discovered upon waking that I would immediately fret about how much time I had left before the alarm went off. I'd look at the clock and calculate the minutes, worrying about how tired I would be if I didn't fall right back to sleep. All this was doing was causing anxiety and releasing cortisol! I do believe in the power of thoughts and decided that nice gentle coaxing about how wonderful it would be to get back into bed and fall asleep would solve the issue. I no longer look at the clock when I wake up, and as long as I don't engage with anyone or anything—especially my thoughts—I do get back into a nice restful slumber.

MODERN STIMULANTS

It is my opinion that modern technological stimulants are the biggest culprit, stealing peaceful rest from everyone who uses them. Not only are they emitting light, not allowing the production of melatonin, but the blue light is very stimulating to the brain. Research shows it takes approximately 90 minutes for your brain to stop processing the blue light after it has been shut down. Proximity to your face plays a role, so the computers, tablets, and phones held right in front of your eyeballs are more detrimental than a television across the room, but that is not recommended either. We also have a tremendous amount of ambient light stymieing melatonin production throughout the night, coming from alarm clocks, nightlights, and the power light on other electronics. The physiological stimulation is just one aspect—think about the cognitive reaction you are having to what you are watching or reading. Is it getting your brain going in a certain way? Is it causing you to release cortisol? If so, this is yet another reason to avoid it before bed.

LIFE AND HORMONAL CYCLES

At various times, hormonal imbalance is a normal part of life, and sleep disturbances may be one side effect. As women cycle through the month, they may notice a few days where they have a harder time sleeping than usual. This is related to the imbalance of estrogen and progesterone. Both of these hormones play key roles—progesterone helping us fall asleep and estrogen helping us stay asleep—and the natural fluctuation can cause disturbance. Similarly, as they enter perimenopause, the dramatic plummet in progesterone production leads many women to have problems with sleep that they never experienced before. This may be cause to consider hormone replacement therapy (always bioidentical and properly dosed and balanced!), because we know the consequences of chronic sleep deprivation are no joke. Low levels of testosterone and a low-functioning thyroid are also connected to poor-quality sleep. As a reminder, I highly suggest the two books, *How to Achieve Healthy Aging* by Dr. Neal Rouzier, and *Stop the Thyroid Madness*, by Janie A. Bowthorpe, M.Ed., to enhance your understanding of hormones before making any decisions on replacement therapy.

SLEEP APNEA

There are roughly twelve million people in the United States with undiagnosed sleep apnea. Apnea literally means "without breath," and sufferers can stop breathing hundreds of times per night. Obstructive sleep apnea is caused by a blockage of the airway, either due to the structure of the throat or when the soft tissue in the back of the throat collapses. With central sleep apnea, the brain fails to signal the muscles to breathe. The rather violent struggle to get oxygen into the body results in loud snoring. Although it seems like just an annoying condition, it should be taken quite seriously. Because you are not able to get deep restful sleep, the activities that take place during Stage 3 and REM are not able to be performed. Health consequences resulting from sleep apnea include memory loss, heart disease, dementia, Alzheimer's, and diabetes. Death is the ultimate consequence most sufferers are in denial about. Each night, without adequate oxygen supply, the heart is required to work harder to circulate what it has, which eventually can result in an enlarged heart. Generally it is the other person in the room who can identify possible sleep apnea, but if you are alone, morning headaches, a dry or sore throat, and feeling tired even after a full night of sleep may indicate the condition. Consult your doctor if you exhibit these symptoms and get involved in a sleep study. In addition to monitoring your movement, you will be connected to a variety of machines measuring brain wave and muscle activity, heart rate, blood pressure, and respiration, which indicate what stage of sleep you are in.

Depending upon the type of sleep apnea—obstructive or central—a variety of treatment options may be available. Excess weight is often a symptom, especially if you have a neck circumference larger than seventeen inches in diameter. Weight loss just might do the trick, but propping up the neck and shoulders can also open the passageway. Sleeping on your side may help, as could a mouth guard. If central sleep apnea is the diagnosis, you will possibly further explore why the message is failing to be sent or delivered. It could indicate a brain stem disorder or could be due to respiratory suppressants, such as from medication or alcohol. The CPAP machine is the last resort for most people, because it is cumbersome and uncomfortable and annoying—but I'd like to think no oxygen is rather annoying as well! I do know that when people who have suffered with sleep apnea finally start getting oxygen throughout the night AND get restful sleep, being a bit uncomfortable is a small price to pay.

NAPS

For many species, human beings included, napping is a normal part of the day. Although some cultures still accommodate the afternoon siesta, most human beings, at least in the United States, do not have the type of schedule that allows for a nap. Ideally your brain would like to rest about 8–10 hours after you've awakened, and because we are overriding the sleepy signal that adenosine is trying to deliver, cortisol is released to help keep you alert and functioning. Sugar and caffeine may be added for an additional boost, only furthering the release of cortisol, which may prevent quality sleep later on. If you are able to sneak away for 20–30 minutes—or even as few as 10—a quick shut-eye can do the trick to get you through your day. You will want to wake up after Stage 2 or sleep a full cycle, or you risk being groggy and more lethargic than prior to your rest!

SLEEP AIDS

Our desire to fix a problem without actually fixing the problem extends to sleep issues. There are countless over-the-counter and prescription sleep aids that will most likely help you sleep, but they could have immediate and long-term side effects. You have probably heard stories from people who take Ambien and may even recall it was used as a defense in a murder trial. Chemicals that tweak our hormones and neurotransmitters are going to cause side effects! The quick fix may lead to bigger problems down the road and is not actually getting to the crux of your sleep issue. Side effects can include elevated blood pressure, elevated blood sugar, night terrors, sleepwalking, and insomnia. Research is showing that long-term, consistent use of antihistamines (the agent in OTC sleep aids) may increase your risk of dementia and Alzheimer's. These are well documented yet readily dismissed, because truly fixing the problem takes work! It's hard. I really encourage you to be well educated on all the ramifications of relying on a sleep aid—then pick your hard.

I think some natural remedies that promote peace and calm can be helpful, but again, these are not miracle solutions. Valerian, lavender, and L-theanine all work on the limbic system—the part of the brain that controls mood. Including these as an overall healthy lifestyle can enhance quality sleep. Melatonin is one of the sleep-inducing hormones, and as we age, production can decline. You may want to consider a low-dose melatonin supplement, but you should still address behaviors that are inhibiting its production, such as inadequate intake of omega-3 fatty acids, ambient light, and electronic device use.

DREAMING

Dreaming is not well understood, but its importance is well recognized. Unless you are truly not getting restful sleep, you are dreaming—even if you don't remember it. Because we spend more time in the REM stage as we get closer to morning, the quantity of sleep is as important as the quality. It appears that the threshold is 6 hours, and any less than that is where we start to see the increased risk for long-term consequences. Some people are very active dreamers; others don't recognize or remember their dreams. There is absolutely no way to determine what the dreams truly mean, but there is plenty of opinion on interpretation. As outlined in Chapter Six, I have always been fascinated by dreams and discovered at a fairly young age that my subconscious is very in tune with my conscious reality. I have learned to not get too wrapped up in what my dreams are trying to tell me specifically but to use them as a barometer for what I may need to address in my awake life. If you feel you want to explore what your subconscious might be trying to push to the surface, my suggestion is to write down the dream as soon as you wake up. Set time aside to reflect on what is going on in your life, generally something that is bothering you. Look for patterns in your dreams, such as a consistent color, setting, or emotion. Sometimes there is symbolic meaning, and other times your dreams are presenting a concern more literally. Determine what steps you can take to put this theme to bed. Do you need to confront the situation, let go of something from your past, or check in on someone you have been out of touch with? Whatever you decide, don't let your dream analysis stress you out! Sometimes it is nothing more than a jumbled mass of thoughts, and if you are struggling to make sense of a dream, it may be best to leave it alone.

IRREGULAR SLEEP SCHEDULE

Those who keep a nontraditional work schedule can face a variety of challenges and perhaps the biggest one is getting adequate sleep. A rotating schedule poses an extra layer of difficulty because the body can never fully adjust to a routine. We know how critical quality sleep is for physical and mental well-being, so taking steps to minimize the impact of this disruption will provide benefits in all aspects of your life. Even in the face of an irregular sleep schedule, taking control and making healthy choices in other areas will reduce these adverse effects and improve your health overall.

Possibly the most important key to successfully transition to more regular sleep is family support. Your schedule will impact everyone around you, so when others understand how important sleep is, hopefully, they will be respectful and supportive of your efforts. Consider a family meeting so everyone knows what the schedule looks like. Be specific about expectations for each family member. Coordination and participation will lead to success, and you may have to gently remind others that when you are well rested, everyone benefits!

Light, both natural and artificial, is the body's cue to wake up. Expose yourself to as much light as possible within 2 hours of waking. If natural light is not available, light therapy using light boxes may be beneficial. Because we need darkness to produce melatonin, try to avoid light when coming off the night shift. Wear dark, wraparound sunglasses when driving home and minimize exposure to any other natural or artificial light, including electronic devices. Melatonin helps the body adjust to its internal clock, so the constant change in your sleep schedule means a supplement is most likely not going to improve your chances of sleep.

A modest amount (200–400 mg) of caffeine may help you wake up and remain alert in the early part of your shift. It should be consumed no later than 6 hours prior to the end of your shift. If you have high blood pressure, you may want to skip it altogether. Alcohol is a major sleep disruptor and ideally should be avoided. Absent any other health conditions, a few adult beverages on your off-days most likely won't harm you, but when heading into or out of a schedule change, remain alcohol free.

Although the sleep schedule is going to change throughout life, keeping a structured sleep pattern is important. Your personal needs, the demands of a job, and requirements on the home front will all play a role in what that pattern looks like. Take time to figure out one that will work for you long term. Your sleep environment should be dark, cool, and quiet. Blackout shades or a sleep mask will help trick your internal clock and facilitate the release of melatonin. Your body temperature fluctuates during the various sleep cycles. A room temperature between 66–68 degrees will prevent you from getting hot and waking up. Quiet or very low white noise is also needed to get into the healing zone of our deep sleep cycles. Creating a separate space for your sleep needs may be necessary. If you have a rotating shift schedule, compromise and creativity will be key. As you are headed into or out of the new schedule, you will want to gradually start adjusting to the new schedule by 1–2 hours each day. This is also a helpful strategy for those who travel across multiple time zones. The number of time zones crossed and the duration of the trip need to be considered, but in my experience, the sooner you participate in the time zone to which your body finds itself, the smoother the transition. For example, when I travel to Hawaii, if the clock says 8:00 p.m., it is 8:00 p.m.—not 11:00 p.m., which it is in Denver. I adjust my routine to go to bed and wake up at the time I want, not the time my body thinks it is based on where I just came from.

I'm sure everyone has had a great night of sleep and truly noticed the difference the next day. Wouldn't it be amazing to feel that way more often? If you struggle with getting quality sleep and are ready to give that struggle a rest, here are some things to consider:

1. Identify the obstacle to sleep (check all that apply)

    - a Busy mind
    - stress (cortisol released throughout the day)
    - inactivity
    - eating too late/types of food/amount of food
    - caffeine (amount and time of day consumed)
    - technology
    - interruptions (kids, animals, full bladder, significant other)
    - other?

2. Create a real strategy to modify a behavior that could be impeding quality sleep.

3. Recognize that it is the cumulative effect of all the things we do consistently over time that has the largest impact on the outcome. Multiple behaviors may need modification, and they have to become your habits to reap the benefits.

FINAL THOUGHTS

The U.S. Centers for Disease Control has officially declared sleep deprivation an epidemic. Through analyzing my own tendencies and acknowledging which ones were potentially impacting my sleep negatively, I have been able to restructure and modify many of those habits. I have an evening wind-down routine, allowing the house, the body, and the mind to get ready for rest. The house gets dark, the body gets relaxed, the mind gets quiet. Although I occasionally have a difficult night of sleep, I am happy to say that insomnia is no longer a regular part of my life. I also know that even though I am doing all I can right now to set myself up for quality sleep, it is not always in my control. I try to make really healthy choices in every other area—what I put in my body, how much I move my body, and how I manage my stress triggers—to, hopefully, minimize the damage that inadequate sleep may be causing. The challenge of setting yourself up for quality sleep may seem like a frustrating and daunting process, but you are a Better Being, one who is ready to take on that challenge. Once I established new habits, the benefits of a better night's rest have allowed me to be a healthier, happier, more productive human being. So far, I have found it worth the effort—and I believe you will too!

Chapter Ten

DECADES

I THINK THERE COMES A time in our lives where we look back and wish we had done a few things differently. I personally wish I would have taken better care of myself in my late teens and early twenties, but at the time, the idea that the choices I was making were actually going to matter at a time other than the immediate future did not even cross my mind. You do what you know, and often you make choices knowing full well they are not good. "I can't help it, this one thing isn't going to matter, I'll worry about it later"—these thoughts were typical and frequent for me. The reality is, I CAN help it, it IS going to matter, and LATER comes sooner than you think!

Human beings are resilient creatures. We first must have awareness that we are causing harm then the desire to stop causing the harm. Each chapter thus far has honed in on behaviors that have a direct or indirect impact on many facets of well-being. I hope you have identified areas for change and determined that you are ready for action. Once we stop causing harm, we need to provide the body and brain resources to heal then continue providing them so we can thrive. This is called the healthy lifestyle.

If you have not yet come to that point in life where you wish you could have a do-over, you are probably part of that amazing group, the YBI—Young, Beautiful, and Invincible. Since nothing is "wrong," why change behaviors? The truth is there may be plenty going wrong; it just hasn't presented itself yet. It's happening, but you just don't know it because you can't see or feel it yet. YET. If you ask people in their forties, fifties, or sixties if they ever thought this would be the outcome, I am willing to bet most would say no. That won't happen to me! I will not end up like my mom, dad, aunt, sister! However, if your habits are similar to what theirs were, the likelihood that you will end up in a similar place is very strong. The sooner we embrace the idea that how we live our daily lives determines how we live our future lives, the better our future lives will be! The good news is it's never too early or too late to make changes in your habits and reap the benefits. Here's a checklist for each decade to keep you engaged and on track so your future self will thank you.

THRIVING THIRTIES

By the time you reach your thirties, you have already gone through many life transitions. You may be noticing changes in energy level, sleep patterns, and ability to maintain a healthy weight. The time to engage is NOW!

KNOW YOUR NUMBERS
Blood pressure
Cholesterol
Blood sugar
Waist circumference

Consistent behaviors have tremendous influence on the outcome. If you are already identifying some potential health issues, educate yourself on what choices you are making that may be increasing your risk for serious consequences in the future. Establish your own personal wellness vision. Create strategies that will help you modify behaviors to achieve that vision. There is no time like the present to instill healthier habits to carry you through life!

OTHER SCREENINGS:
Pelvic/Testicular exam
Skin cancer screening
Vision
Dental
Flu shots

FIERCE FORTIES
The forties bring many changes in all facets of life. You may be sandwiched in the middle of caring for kids as well as your aging parents. You are struggling to balance career, family, and your own health. The stressors of life are starting to be reflected in your physical and mental well-being.

This may be a great time to establish new boundaries and to learn how to say no. Make your health a priority—make your-SELF a priority!

By now we all know that nutrition, movement, stress management, and sleep are critical for overall health and wellness. You may notice the weight comes on quickly and barely budges when you try to "be good." You may want to blame it on your metabolism, but it is a myth that metabolism drops simply as a function of age. Follow these steps to boost yours:

Eat more (real food!)
Drink more (water)

Lift more ("heavy" weight)
Sleep more (minimum seven hrs)
Sprint more (high-intensity cardio)

In addition to the screenings of your thirties, it may be time for a mammogram. You also might want to think about getting hormone levels tested including:

Full thyroid panel
Cortisol
Estrogen/Progesterone/Testosterone

FABULOUS FIFTIES

If you haven't already noticed, your hormone levels are dropping! We are not supposed to be able to procreate forever, and the decline in the production of our sex hormones is in place for just that reason. However, we are now living well past childbearing years, and as outlined in the book *How to Achieve Healthy Aging* by Dr. Neal Rouzier, balanced hormones at optimal levels keep us healthy and thriving. Consider getting your levels tested to determine if bioidentical replacement therapy could provide symptom relief, enhanced health, and improved well-being.

For women, perimenopause is that phase of life lasting anywhere from one to ten years. There is a rather rapid reduction of all sex hormones, and it is the dramatic drop in progesterone that largely determines your menopause experience. Less than adequate levels of testosterone in women can also contribute to symptoms. The book *What's Your Menopause Type?* by Joseph Collins, N.D., is a great resource for helping you navigate through this transitional time in life. The ratios of the hormones involved—estrogen, progesterone, and testosterone—influence the symptoms and health risks. There are twelve possible combinations, which is why women can have very different experiences, and why different treatments are better for some than others. Once women are through menopause, marked by one full year with no menses, many symptoms diminish, but health risks may increase. Estrogen keeps our hearts, brains, and bones healthy, and with decreased production of it comes an increased risk for heart disease, memory issues, and bone loss. If you have health risks going into menopause, you will have greater risk after menopause, so take charge of your choices.

Men also go through a drop in hormone production, but it is more gradual over several decades. "Manopause" symptoms and complications from decreased testosterone include thinning hair, increased body fat, loss of muscle mass, and decreased libido. Men may be at increased risk for sleep apnea, declining cognitive function, and depression. Bioidentical replacement therapy is an option for boosting testosterone to optimal levels for enhanced well-being into later years.

In addition to the regular screenings, it's also time for a bone density test, a colonoscopy, and a prostate exam.

SUPER SIXTIES

Retirement is near—are you ready? We all know being financially prepared is necessary, but are you mentally ready for this new phase of life?

Learn a new skill, volunteer, work part time, hone a hobby, exercise! Whatever you do, don't sit still. Stay physically, mentally, and socially engaged to enjoy these years you have worked so hard for. Maintaining some type of structure to your schedule will help keep you accountable and on track with healthy choices.

In addition to regular screenings, include a shingles vaccine and a hearing test.

MY FINAL FINAL THOUGHTS

We have come to the end . . . of the book, not the journey! It is with deep gratitude that I thank you for taking the time to enter my world. I hope you were informed, inspired, and a bit entertained. Perhaps your mind is in overdrive, flooded with ideas of changes you want to make in your life. Maybe you are a little deflated at the prospect of all the changes you NEED to make in your life. Whatever you are feeling, take a deep breath. You ARE a Better Being. You have everything you need to begin or continue your journey to living the life you desire and deserve. I, too, will continue on my journey, as I know there is still plenty of room for growth and improvement. As I move through the rest of my life, I will do so with a set of intentions, and I will close out our time together by sharing them with you.

Aloha always and in all ways,

Michelle

INTENTIONS OF A BETTER BEING

I will practice patience.

I will be kind to myself and others.

I will nourish my brain and body with high-quality fuel.

I will honor my body's need for movement.

I will work on letting go of the things
I cannot change or control.

I will withhold judgment if I don't
know the whole story.

I will strive to make better choices
today than I did yesterday.

I will acknowledge my strengths and use
them to address my weaknesses.

I will identify my obstacles and work to create
strategies around them.

I will accept the fact that there is no such thing
as an instant result with no effort.

I will embrace my journey with an open
mind and a positive attitude.

REFERENCE SHEETS

NUTRITION CATEGORIES

FIBER—AKA CARBS—40-45% OF TOTAL DAILY CALORIES

Most of your servings of carbohydrate should be vegetables, and you should aim for every color of the rainbow among your fruits and vegetables.

Vegetables
- All types of lettuce EXCEPT iceberg
- Spinach
- Broccoli
- Cauliflower
- All varieties of peppers
- Onions
- Green beans
- Asparagus
- Brussels sprouts

- Eggplant
- Mushrooms
- Carrots
- Sweet potatoes, purple sweet potatoes, and yams
- Zucchini
- Squash

Fruits

- Tomatoes
- Berries of all types
- Apples
- Pears
- Bananas
- Oranges
- Melons of all types
- Pineapples
- Mangoes
- Figs
- Dates

Grains, Beans, Legumes, Seeds

- Whole grains—wheat, oat, barley, millet, bulger—also have a bit of protein
- Quinoa—actually a seed but acts like a grain—also has protein
- Brown rice
- All types of beans and legumes—also have protein
- Seeds—also have protein and fat

PROTEIN—25-30% OF TOTAL DAILY CALORIES

- All meats—also possibly has fat depending on the type and cut of meat

- Fish—salmon, herring, sardines, mackerel have healthy fat; other are a lean source of protein

- Eggs—also have fat

- Dairy—Greek yogurt is best source—others can have a considerable amount of sugar and not as much protein

- Beans—black, navy, white, garbanzo—also have fiber

- Nuts and nut butters—also have fat and fiber

- Seeds—flax, chia, sesame, sunflower—also have fat and fiber

- Legumes—also have fiber

- Soy and soy products—also have fiber

- Protein powders—whey, soy, pea, hemp, plant variety

FAT—25-30% OF TOTAL DAILY CALORIES

- Avocados—also has fiber
- Olive oil
- Coconut oil
- Almond oil
- Avocado oil
- High-Oleic sunflower -il
- Butter
- Lard
- Tallow (beef fat)
- Fatty fish
- Dairy foods—milk, cheese, yogurt, cottage cheese—also

have protein
- Seeds—chia, hemp, pumpkin, sunflower, ground flax—also have protein and fiber
- Nuts and nut butters—also have protein and fiber

MICHELLE'S FAVORITE PFF COMBOS

- Hard-boiled egg and a Granny Smith apple

- Veggies of ALL kinds roasted in olive or avocado oil with some type of meat

- My oatmeal: 1/3 cup oats; 1 Tbsp. ground flax seeds; ½ banana; 1/3 cup walnuts, cinnamon, or pumpkin spice; ½ cup unsweetened almond or coconut milk and water

- ½ cup plain nonfat Greek yogurt with 1 Tbsp. low-sugar chocolate protein powder, and ¼ cup blueberries

- 1 slice whole grain toast with my homemade nut butter (almond-walnut mix with coconut oil). Sometimes I add a few banana slices or butter. Butter on nut butter is DELISH!

- Egg Scramble: Every vegetable you like (spinach, mushrooms, onions, tomatoes, all colors of peppers, and shaved Brussels sprouts) sautéed in avocado oil. Scramble eggs through and add avocado and/or a bit of feta cheese. Wrap it up in a whole grain tortilla if you need a bit more carbohydrate.

- Asparagus and riced cauliflower roasted with olive oil served with seasoned fish (halibut and mahi-mahi are my favorites).

- Smoothies—PFF! Think any ingredients and flavors you like, but make sure you have plenty of protein and fat; greens; and some fruit (but not too much!); Greek yogurt or protein powder for the protein; and coconut oil, avocado, nuts or nut butter, chia or ground flax seeds for the fat. One of my favorites is plain Greek yogurt, chocolate protein powder, unsweetened coconut milk, ½ frozen banana, 2 cups spinach, 2 Tbsp. nut butter, and a dash of cinnamon.

- Veggies with hummus—SO many yummy varieties to try so you will never get bored! I usually have a few of Mary's Gone Crackers with them as well.

- Thinly sliced Lacey Swiss cheese, with toasted chicken, avocado, and fresh ground pepper all rolled up.

- Spinach Salad: spinach, hard-boiled egg, thinly sliced apple, feta cheese, hemp seeds, slivered almonds, and my homemade dressing of avocado oil and balsamic vinegar.

- Granny Smith apple with goat cheese and walnuts with a drizzle of balsamic vinegar.

- Lazy Burrito: On a whole grain tortilla, place some refried beans, fresh salsa, and a bit of extra sharp cheddar. Microwave for 45 seconds and add fresh avocado and plain Greek yogurt as a sour cream substitute.

- Brussels sprouts or green beans sautéed in avocado oil with white onion and mushrooms—add feta or fresh grated Parmesan cheese for next-level deliciousness.

ACKNOWLEDGMENTS

How does one properly acknowledge all the people who have been so influential in my life? I'm not really sure, but here's my best attempt.

Mom and Dad. When it comes to parents, I hold the golden ticket. From the start, you supported and nurtured my independence. When I wanted to participate in gymnastics, instead of school sports and Brownies like all my friends, you said, "OK." When I wanted to paint my VW Bug hot pink, you said, "Bring me the color." When I told you I was going to go to school in Hawaii, we negotiated a few parameters then you made it happen. I know I was not the easiest child, and an even more difficult teenager, but, hopefully, I have made up for it as your adult daughter. Your constant dedication to each other and to us as a family is truly the best gift a girl can receive. Your love, support, patience, guidance, help, and sacrifice have made my journey the best it could possibly be. I love you both for everything you do and everything you are.

Nicolle. I concede it wasn't easy having me as a sister, but I know our relationship would not be what it is today if not for all those testy times. Thank you for never giving up on our sistership, putting me in check when I deserved it and your patience when I didn't. You have become my biggest cheerleader and a friend I truly enjoy spending time with. We have so much ahead of us, and I am excited to see what adventures we will share. Love you lots, Sister.

Phyllis and Dale. For a great period of my life, I spent more time with you than any other people. I will never forget the love I felt the first time I saw you after I quit the team. I was terrified to face you, but you embraced me with compassion. You have influenced the lives of thousands of girls, and although we all have different experiences, I am forever grateful for mine. The lessons you taught me, whether intentionally or inadvertently, have carried me through many facets<<mean phases? of my life. I treasure the times we have been able to connect over the past thirty years and look forward to many more.

My childhood friends. Although I am no longer close to most, you may be surprised at how often you are on my mind (and in my dreams!). I am now a big city girl, but our little class of 106 fit me perfectly back then. These are my roots, and I treasure the memories of growing up in small town Wisconsin. A special shout-out to Jesica and her beautiful family of husband Andy (also a classmate and my prom date!) and children Grace, John, MaryKate, and Andrew. It is no small feat to run the King household AND tend to a long-distance friend, but through the years, our friendship has only become stronger. I thank you for the effort and look forward to many years of continued friendship and to my role as Fun Aunt Michelle.

Adulthood friends. Through thick and thin (literally and figuratively), you have been there.

Lisa. From my first days in Hawaii at the Atherton, it was clear you would be a huge influence in my life. You were my first big city friend, and twenty-seven years later I am grateful you are still by my side (and a mere four miles away). I may have pushed us through the Honolulu Marathon, but you have always challenged me to think bigger, be more, do better. Our rich history of laughter, tears, shenanigans, and banana pancakes far exceeds the challenging moments we endured, and whatever the future holds, I know it will be great because you are my friend. I cannot adequately express how much I appreciate all you have done to encourage, support, and celebrate me. Aloha and mahalo my friend.

Kelly. Who is this seventeen-year-old bottle of energy who barreled into my life? This is what I thought twenty-seven years ago when you finally decided to show up at school. Although that stay was brief, oh, what fun we had! You left a huge mark on my heart, and the following years you were there for some of my toughest times. The love and support (and casseroles) you offered will never be forgotten. Our friendship has grown in so many ways, but you'll always be my little Kell Bell. So much lies ahead for both of us, and I am excited to see what the next twenty-seven years looks like!

Martha. The cliché "everything happens for a reason" rings true for me. Out of a doomed relationship came a beautiful friendship, and all the grief I endured with David was totally worth it! Thank you, my friend, for always having me in your prayers and for continuing to nurture our long-distance friendship. I especially enjoy our conversations while we are both driving to appointments. Whether we get to talking about a personal or professional issue, I come away with something positive. I look forward to entering the next phase of our lives and to continuing our new tradition of a yearly girls trip!

Jen. The day you walked out of our training session because I had you on the StairMaster was a very sad day for me. THANK YOU for coming back! It is crazy to think we are nearing twenty years of friendship—and what a wild bunch of years they have been. Neither of us could have predicted all that has transpired, and who knows what's in store for the next twenty. I'm sure they will be book worthy! I admire and love you, my friend.

Jim and Sandy. How did I get so lucky to find some of the best Wisconsin friends in little old Gunbarrel, Colorado?! More than twenty years of friendship stem from those early days at the gym when you immediately welcomed me as a member of your family. No matter what, I can always count on you for love, laughs, and ridiculously in-depth Packers knowledge! I am forecasting lots of wins for all of us.

Brandon. Your light burns brighter than any other I know. It may not be obvious, but I feel truly blessed to be in the sphere of your glow. You call me your mentor, but I have learned as much, if not more, by being in your presence. Great things await as you continue to shine. Thank you for sharing your light with me.

To all those I have encountered along the way, whether knowingly or not, you have challenged me to be a Better Being. I am grateful for each experience and look forward to the many more that lie ahead.

I have an abundance of gratitude for all those who have given me opportunities in my professional pursuits. Better Beings, the business, certainly would not have flourished without the continued support of many professional alliances. Thank you all for allowing me to live my passion and make a living while doing so! A special thanks to Tanya and Lori, for having faith in my knowledge and ability to create a program that would not only challenge those who participated but also challenge me to grow and develop professionally. I could not have imagined the impact that a single opportunity would have on so many lives or that it would eventually be the impetus for writing a book. I am eternally grateful for your belief in me back then and your continued support.

When I decided to write this book, I knew I'd need time and space without distractions to get it done. What I could never have imagined is that I would stumble upon Tammy L. Coia, The Memoir Coach. A random Internet search led me to make one of the best decisions of my life: to take a private writing retreat with you in Bellingham, Washington. I can't thank you enough for the environment you shared, which allowed me to accomplish more than I could possibly have imagined in those three days. The subtle tribute to Hawaii, where my soul lives; the constant, and I mean CONSTANT, supply of delicious healthy food; and your loving creatures, Bruce and Sophia, serving as cheerleaders and accountability coaches—all contributed to my motivation and creative flow. Your guidance, encouragement, and friendship are so greatly valued, and the fact that you are a die-hard Packers fan elevates you even more. I love experiencing what I teach . . . that when we set ourselves up for success with a supportive and nurturing environment, proper fuel, solid rest, and a dash of fun, we will thrive. Eight short months ago I didn't know where this would land. Thank you for all you have done to help it officially come to life.

I have been moved by the enthusiastic encouragement dished out by so many throughout this process. In particular, thanks to

Stephanie, Renee, Kit, Tahverlee, Jody, Beth, Ruth, and Maribeth for keeping close tabs on the progress and generously offering your ears and arms when I needed some sorting out.

A Better Being knows when to spend time and energy to figure something out and when to hand it off to the experts. Enter Polly Letofsky at My Word Publishing. You assembled an incredible team that was with me every step of the way. Thank you, Bobby, Victoria, and Angela for your patience with this rookie writer and for turning my vision and thoughts into a published piece of work! Thank you, Polly, for your support, encouragement, and dedication to the details of this project. I could have done it without you, but it would have been MUCH more difficult, and not nearly as much fun!

ABOUT THE AUTHOR

The seeds for Michelle Zellner's career in wellness were planted at age seven when she excelled as a gymnast. After devoting her childhood to competition, she hung up the grips to attend the University of Hawaii and earn her B.A. in psychology with a minor in nutrition. Shortly after, she completed an M.S. in kinesiology with a sports psychology emphasis. Michelle quickly discovered the beauty of combining all of her passions into a business, and she created Better Beings. Her formula Better Minds + Better Bodies = Better Beings sums it up nicely.

Michelle now motivates, inspires, and empowers others all over the country to embrace a healthy lifestyle through her Better Beings wellness programs. If you would like Michelle to ignite your group with a keynote speech, corporate training, or custom-designed weekend workshop, please contact her through www.betterbeings.net.

Connect with Michelle:
betterbeingsus
@betterbeingsus